the Red Record

THE WALLAM OLUM

The Oldest Native North American History

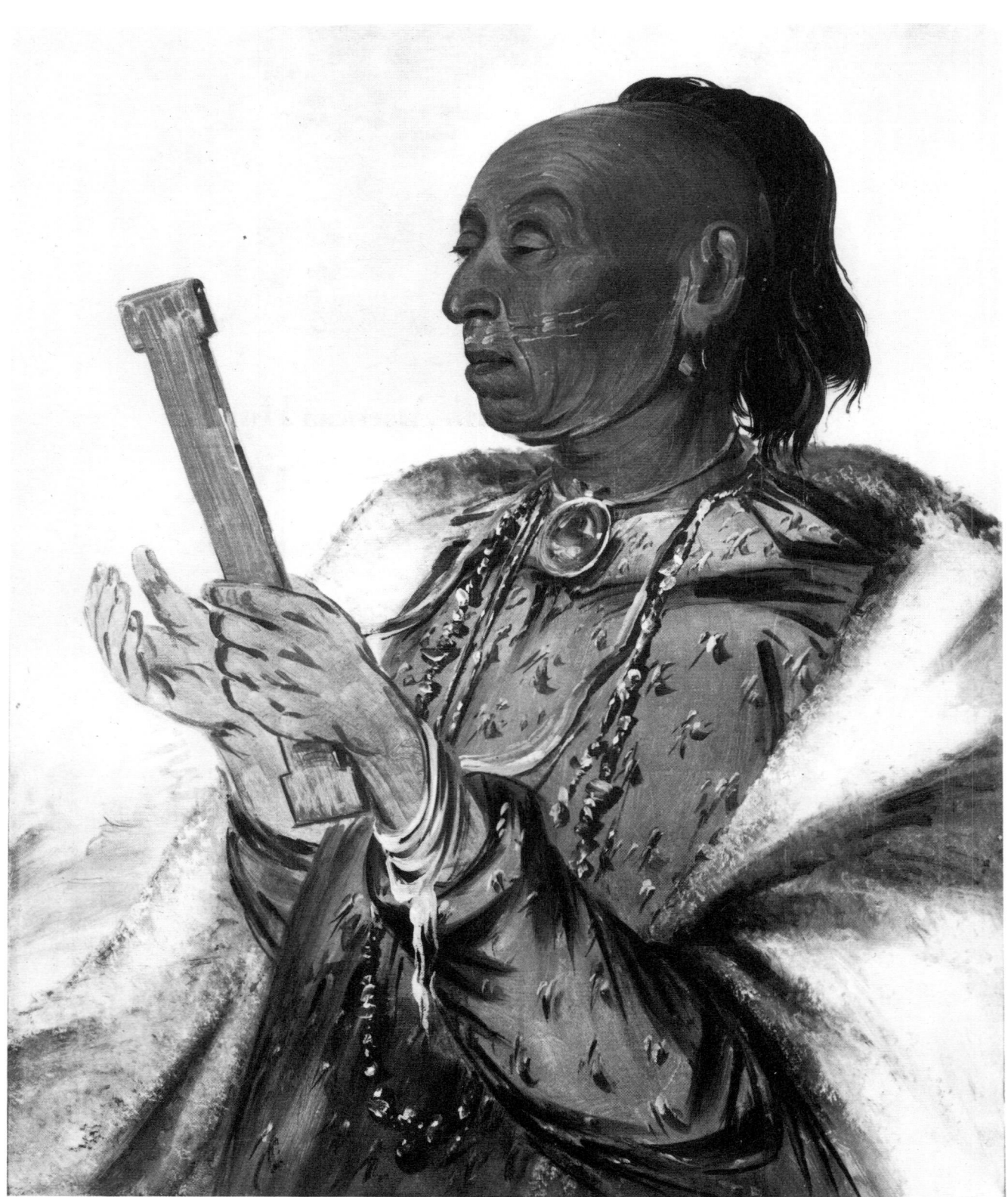

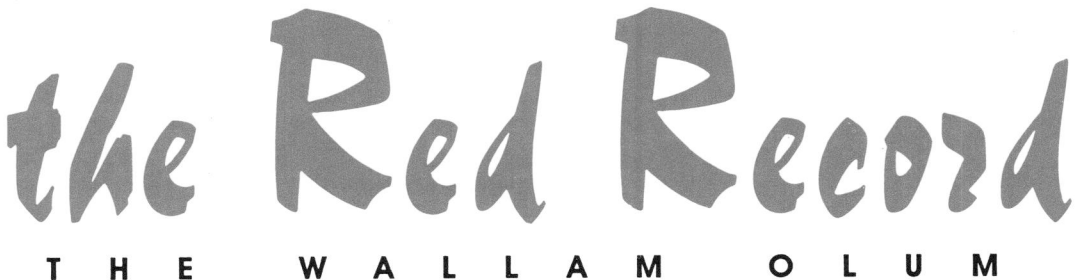

the Red Record

THE WALLAM OLUM

The Oldest Native North American History

TRANSLATED AND ANNOTATED BY

David McCutchen

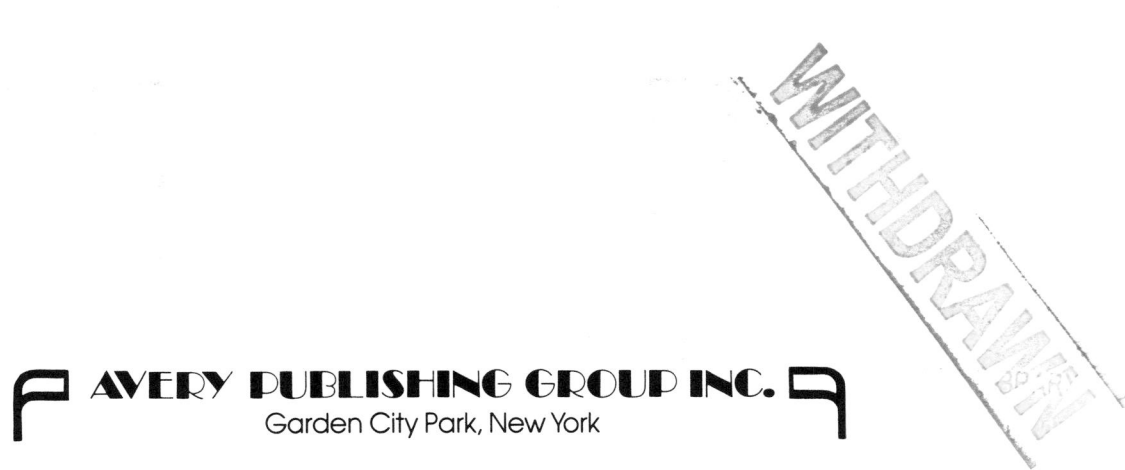

AVERY PUBLISHING GROUP INC.
Garden City Park, New York

Cover Designers: Rudy Shur and Ann Vestal
Cover Photograph: Desert Ridges, Penaleno Mountains, AZ
© 1989 David Muench
Original Artwork: David McCutchen
In-House Editor: Linda Comac
Typesetter: Bonnie Freid

Frontispiece. The frontispiece depicts Cock Turkey, a Kickapoo, reciting from a prayer stick, as painted by George Catlin in 1830. The Kickapoos were relatives of the Delawares; this man's appearance probably resembles that of the Delaware historian who first read the Red Record to Dr. Ward in 1820 from wooden tablets such as those in the painting. (Courtesy of National Museum of American Art, Smithsonian Institution. Gift of Mrs. Joseph Harrison, Jr.)

Library of Congress Cataloging-in-Publication Data

Wallam Olum. English.
    The red record : the Wallam olum of the Lenni Lenape, the Delaware
Indians, a translation and study / by David McCutchen : illustrated
by the author.
        p.   cm.
    Includes bibliographical references and index.
    ISBN 0-89529-525-3 : $14.95
        1. Delaware Indians—History.   2. Delaware Indians—Legends.
    3. Delaware language—Texts.   4. Delaware Indians—Writing.
    I. McCutchen, David.   II. Title
    E99'.D2W2413 1993
    973'.04973—dc20   92-23247
                                                                         CIP

10 9 8 7 6 5 4 3 2 1

Contents

*For those who have seen America today
and wondered what it was like . . . Before*

Acknowledgments

I would like to thank Dr. Gregory Schaaf, who first introduced me to the Wallam Olum and to the Lenni Lenape, and who has guided and advised me throughout the writing of this book. No other tribe has been so extensively documented over such a long period of time as the Delawares, and the sheer volume of material from their rich history can sometimes be overwhelming. But Greg always managed to plunge into the mass and fish out something that would answer our questions. Without his aid and encouragement, this book would not have been possible.

Rudy Shur and Linda Comac of Avery have been invaluable in helping to shape the mass of material in this book into a well-designed form, and in finding ways to communicate the essentials of a complex subject with grace and clarity.

I would also like to thank the Delawares of Oklahoma, especially Linda Poolaw of Anadarko and Henry and Belva Secondine of Bartlesville. They were more than helpful to Greg and me and showed that the traditions of the Lenni Lenape still live on today. Whatever happens, the Delawares will endure, and prevail.

Finally I would like to thank the many scholars, living and dead, who have worked to add to our understanding of the Wallam Olum and this important Native American culture. I am especially grateful to Paul Weer for his research into how the Wallam Olum first came into the hands of white people and what became of the original documents, and to the devoted Moravian missionary Reverend John Heckewelder, who did so much to preserve the history and traditions of the people he lived among and loved.

Foreword

It seems as though the Delaware or Lenni Lenape have been on the North American continent forever. I remember hearing legends and myths from my elders describing prehistoric animals and people. These awesome stories would keep me awake on hot summer nights or cold winter evenings. My imagination would take me back into the distant past, to encounters with extinct animals, and I could see the vision of a giant turtle with children on its back entering the ocean. I would wonder how it would be to live near the "big water."

How and what we learned had been taught to our parents and to their parents before them. Since so many things had to be remembered and recalled, selected people were responsible for selected subjects. The older people or Grandparents were almost always used for this task. Long after these people would go to their final resting place, I could still hear their voices. Even as an adult, I find some parts of their stories still enter my dreams at night.

Once, while visiting a respected Lenape teacher, I mistakenly asked the word, "Why?" I was immediately scolded and told that I sounded just like a "sha-wa-nuk" or "White Person" because "White People" are always asking "why this" or "why that." The teacher instructed me to be like my clan, The Turtle. "Just listen; it takes the turtle a long time to get somewhere, but it knows where it has been. Listen!!"

That is very hard to do in this world. Almost no one listens. My modern education has taught me to ask questions and hurry to get the answers. But since I have made the decision to live by the traditions of my people, the Lenape, I have tried to take the teacher's advice. I can imagine if I were a turtle and had to crawl all the way from the East Coast where the Lenape once lived to where I live now, I would be very wise.

David McCutchen has listened, too. From his earliest encounters with the Wallam Olum, he was able to hear the voices of the Grandfathers, voices that would lead him through years of work, toward the meaning of the ancient symbols and language. With the artist's ability to perceive what is not always apparent to others, David has achieved a remarkable, and, I believe, accurate translation of the Red Record. In David's book, we return again to the days of my ancestors, to the time when their myths and legends were born. Here, in terms a modern audience can appreciate, the story is told anew, of how carefully accumulated experience, guided by respect for tradition and harmony with the environment, can create a living, growing culture.

The Wallam Olum, I believe, conveys such a message. It is an old song, by an ancient people. I believe it was sung by the Grandfathers. I believe it was sung many, many times for many, many centuries. I believe it was sung by my ancestors, as they traveled thousands of miles in search of that place where the Sun wakes up. I pray that this song of the Lenape will be heard. Listen.

Linda Poolaw
Grand Chief
Delaware Nation Grand Council of North America, Inc.
Anadarko, Oklahoma

Preface

I n the spring of 1976, my friend Gregory Schaaf was studying for his doctorate in history at the University of California at Santa Barbara, when he happened upon what the *Los Angeles Times* called "the historical find of the bicentennial." The "find," a previously unknown collection of documents from George Morgan, the first American Indian Agent, detailed how and why the key Native American tribes in 1776 chose not to oppose the fledgling American Revolution. Greg, who has gone on to become a nationally recognized authority on Indian affairs, invited me to join in his research to learn more about the Native Americans who had played such a crucial role in the birth of the United States, protecting it during its most vulnerable period.

As we learned more about the Native American tribal nations that held the balance of power on the frontier in the 1770s, it became clear that the situation then was the result of even earlier events, before the European colonists had arrived, when the Native American nations were the only powers on this continent. The relationships established among the Native Americans in this earliest time extended into colonial times, and determined crucial alliances and family relationships. In the intricate political web of tribes in the Eastern Woodlands, stretching from the East Coast into the Midwest, one group stood out as the kingpins that held alliances together, a group that commanded respect, and therefore was able to speak for large numbers of the tribes. This group was the Lenni Lenape or Delaware Indians. Through their visionary chief, White Eyes, these Native American "Founding Fathers" were able to establish an equal relationship with the new Continental Congress, and win approval, in one of the first United States-Indian treaties, for the idea of a fourteenth state for Indians, a state in which the Delawares would have played a leading role.

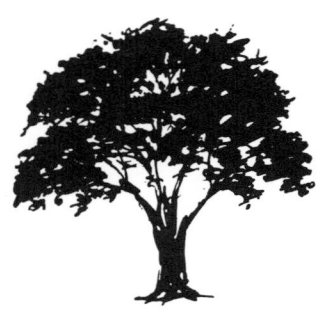

The Shackamaxon elm.
Tradition says that the Great Treaty was concluded beneath the "tree of peace" in Shackamaxon, now part of Philadelphia.

The prestige of the Delawares stemmed from their valor and diplomatic skills, as well as from their heritage. Colonial records are full of tales of their noble and generous conduct, including one of the few completely successful Indian-European agreements, the Great Treaty with William Penn. In searching for the sources of the spiritual strength of the Delawares, we became aware of how their pride came from a deep sense of their roots, the knowledge that they were descended from a long line of heroes.

One day Greg brought home from the library a large, beautifully bound volume full of scholarly notations and pictures of a faded manuscript filled with symbols and unfamiliar words. This was a copy of the landmark Indiana Historical Society study of the Wallam Olum—the Red Record. A Delaware chronicle, it describes in symbols and words, the ancient days before the colonists came, and is the only surviving history of pre-Columbian times north of Mexico.

I was astonished that such an account existed. I wondered why I had never heard of it. I knew that no knowledge of American history could be complete without knowing this original story of how Native Americans came to know this land, a story told from the point of view of one of the leading tribes in North America.

I wanted to know more. At first glance the account appeared cryptic, enigmatic, full of unexplained hints and references. Then the scholarly explanations in the book and elsewhere began to fill in the missing pieces, and I could see the outlines of a story of vast scope, a multi-generational adventure spanning a virgin continent. There were names and events, heroes and villains, travels from arctic wastes into deep forests, as the Delawares, then known as the Lenni Lenape, spread and flourished and produced a mighty national family.

The Lenni Lenape and their relatives were among the first to encounter the European colonists. Historical descriptions of them by the Europeans pick up almost without a break from the time when the Wallam Olum ends. So by adding European, colonial, and American records to the information in the Wallam Olum, we can see a continuous description, covering more than a thousand years, of the life of at least one Native American tribe north of Mexico.

Greg and I began to conceive of a narrative based on this idea, a kind of Native American *Roots*, featuring a succession of Delaware heroes continuing a heritage that reached back, deep into this continent's past. Since he specialized in the Lenape story as recorded in colonial records, Greg wrote about the period leading up to and beyond the American Revolution. I concentrated on the "prehistoric" times described in the Wallam Olum.

I began trying to read the Wallam Olum as a narrative, looking for a logical series of events that could be revealed through its cryptic clues. I quickly became frustrated by the obscurities and contradictions of existing translations, which seemed arbitrary and lacking in sense in English. So I undertook to create an improved translation, based upon years of research into Delaware language, culture, historical traditions, and legends. This research led to a clearer picture of what the Wallam Olum says, and what it means. I also uncovered unexpected evidence of the Wallam Olum's accuracy, and of when and how it was composed.

Research also revealed that although almost universally accepted as a genuine Delaware production, the Wallam Olum is dismissed by some as mere legends, unsupported by facts. This is what used to be said about the *Iliad*, before excavations by Heinrich Schliemann showed that Troy actually existed. But do his findings prove that there was ever a person named Achilles? Ancient names and deeds are almost impossible to confirm, even with the best of records. There are skeptics who doubt the existence even of Moses and Jesus.

Even when events are described in writing, there will be controversy about whether or not they are true. Lawyers, journalists, and historians constantly battle over what is fact and what is fiction, and not everyone will be satisfied. We may never know how much of the Wallam Olum is fact and how much is fiction; how much is accurate and how much might have been garbled or lost in transmission. What is important is for the Wallam Olum to be acknowledged as a possible, if shadowy, beginning of our written history, like the Norse sagas of Leif Erikson's voyages to America.

No other Native American account north of Mexico extends so far back into the past, or includes such a wealth of historical detail. It seems to extend back at least as far as the pre-Columbian times of such Central American civilizations as the Maya. Just how far back the Wallam Olum extends is difficult to say, since the Lenni Lenape did not develop a calendar or a written system of dates because they did not share the modern obsession with what the Maya called "the burden of time." In any event, because of the comprehensiveness of its descriptions, the Wallam Olum is entitled to a position of pre-eminence in American history. Its place in the annals of history is further enhanced by its being the oldest Native American history, especially if "Native American" is understood to refer to the tribes of what is now the United States and Canada. This situation is similar to "America" being generally understood to refer to the United States alone, although technically the word can include the rest of North America and South America as well.

The vagueness and ambiguity with which the Wallam Olum has been presented in the past have prevented a general audience from understanding it. But seen in the right light, the Wallam Olum can come to life and become a vivid part of our national experience. This book is an effort to clear up some of the confusion surrounding the interpretation of the Wallam Olum, and to turn it from an academic curio into a piece of living history.

Because the Wallam Olum is very condensed in form, some explanation must accompany it. This book, therefore, introduces the Wallam Olum with an examination of its significance, a look at how it describes time and place, and an introduction to the native culture that produced it. Then, following a brief note on how the original record tablets were reconstructed, the words and symbols of the Wallam Olum are presented, with a new translation, divided into chapters representing the probable original divisions of the symbols onto separate tablets. On a facing page, each chapter is given a descriptive title, with annotations and explanations. A number of chapters include original illustrations and maps showing the apparent locations for many of the events described in the story.

This ends the section presenting the Lenni Lenape records of the time before the coming of the European colonists. But the story does not end here. Using other sources, we can continue to hear, in the words of the Lenni Lenape, a Native American view of American history. Part Two, therefore, ends at the point of transition from the conclusion of the Wallam Olum to contemporary times, with the fascinating Lenni Lenape account of their first meeting with European explorers.

The story as told by the Lenni Lenape, later known as the Delawares, is then continued into the nineteenth century by the "Fragment"—a historical document that gives a native view of the major events of Delaware life from the end of the Wallam Olum in 1620 to their westward crossing of the Mississippi in 1820. This native account is presented with appropriate explanations and annotations.

The book concludes with a brief account of the Delawares' later history up to the present day, and a look at the Wallam Olum in comparison to other ancient legends and historical traditions from around the world. I hope that this will stimulate a renewed appreciation for the Wallam Olum, the culture that produced it, and the country where it took place.

A Note on Terminology

Confronted with an alien culture, explorers, colonists, and scientists grope for words to describe what they have found. The choices of terms made in those first descriptions can be unfortunate because they often endure even if they are inaccurate. The naming of Native Americans as "Indians" by Columbus is just one example. The subject matter of this book has been given so many distorted names that, in order to prevent further misconceptions, a brief redefinition of terms is necessary.

First of all, "Delaware Indians" is a name given them by outsiders. The original name of the Delawares was the "Lenni Lenape," the "Original People," which has also been variously translated as the "True People," "People People," "Men of Men," and even "We, the People." In 1610, Captain Samuel Argall sailed up their river and named it and the people who lived along it after his patron, Lord De La Warr, or Delaware for short. Because 1610 also roughly marks the point at which the Wallam Olum ends and the "modern age" begins, this book will refer to the people as the "Lenni Lenape" in the story that takes place before 1610, and as the "Delawares" thereafter. This latter name, as we have seen, stems from the Delaware River, not the state of that name; although the tribe lived in that state, its main settlements were in what is now known as New Jersey and Pennsylvania.

To add to the distortion, the great national family of the Lenni Lenape has been misnamed the Algonquians (also called the Algonquin or the Algonkins) after a small tribe in Canada, as if the Delawares were descended from them, instead of vice versa. Because so many of the Algonquian tribes were proud to trace their roots to the Lenni Lenape or "Grandfathers," I will call them the Lenape family of tribes, so here the terms "Lenape" and "Algonquian" can be understood to be interchangeable. Since the Wallam Olum is apparently a record kept by a core group of the Lenape-Algonquians, the events it describes can be understood as representative of the general actions of all or most of the Lenape family.

When referring to both Lenape and non-Lenape native people together, I use "Native Americans," if possible, or "Indians" if that reflects a more common usage, as in "Indian Agent."

The Wallam Olum, as well as the people, has suffered from misdescription. There is not even a commonly accepted spelling for the name. At various times, it has been called the Walum Olum, Walam Olum, Wallamolum, Olum Wolum, and Wallam-olum. I use the spelling most often used in the Rafinesque Manuscript, the earliest surviving record of the Wallam Olum. As for the translation of the name, that too has varied widely because the words have many shades of meaning. Rather than give a literal reading of the name—"Ancient Fine-Looking (painted sacred-color-Red) Engraved Tally-Score-Record"—I will simply call it the Red Record.

Part One

Echoes of Ancient Voices

Chapter One

A Key to Prehistory

Long before the great cities of glass and steel arose along the Eastern Seaboard of the United States, the area was the homeland of another nation, a Native American nation, with its own traditions, its own history, and its own past heroes. The European invasion that began with Columbus shattered this nation and swept it away, but it left behind a record of that history to give us a last glimpse of Ancient America.

This account is called the Wallam Olum, the Red Record, and the people who wrote it are the Lenni Lenape, later named the "Delaware Indians." After a twenty-year study of the Red Record, the Indiana Historical Society pronounced it "probably the most important and most interesting recorded tradition derived from any aboriginal source north of Mexico."[1]

The aboriginal source of the Red Record, the Lenni Lenape, or "Original People," were widely known and respected among the Indian tribes. With a deep knowledge of their past and a tradition of pictographic records, the Lenni Lenape were uniquely qualified to write this chronicle of ancient heroes and events. As the anthropologist Werner Muller notes:

In the long chain of tribes along the East Coast, one ethnic group stands out, not only in the European written sources but also in the judgement of the Indians themselves. This remarkable group was the Delaware, called in their own language the Lenni Lenape. They had a special status in the eyes of many other Indian peoples: they were reverenced as the 'grandfathers,' representatives, after a fashion, of authority and legality.[2]

The Wallam Olum, the Red Record, is the Delawares' record of their ancient history, told in the form of an epic song. Recorded in pictures and words, the saga tells of the rise to glory of the Lenni Lenape and their great Lenape family, also called the Algonquians, the most populous and widespread Native American language group in ancient North America. The Delawares today firmly believe that this is the record of their past. The Delaware tribal Business Committee, meeting in Bartlesville, Oklahoma, recently called the Red Record tablets "the ancient tribal record tablets of our ancestors, the Lenni Lenape."[3] And the Delaware elder Winnie Poolaw of Anadarko, Oklahoma, declared, "The Wallam Olum is like our Bible."[4]

The Red Record begins with the Lenape accounts of Creation and of a great Flood. It then tells of the crossing of the Lenape people from Asia into the New World, and of their encounters with the people who were already living there. It goes on to recount the epic journey of the Lenape south and eastward across North America, and the succession of sachems or chiefs who led them. Nearly one hundred generations of these leaders are described, an unbroken chain of names and deeds stretching over thousands of years and thousands of miles. Along the way, the Lenape people survive divisions, droughts, and wars to find a happy ending in a homeland centered in the beautiful Delaware River Valley. The Red Record ends with a description of the arrival of European ships on the Delaware River around 1620:

Friendly people, in great ships; who are they?

The Lenni Lenape and their Lenape relatives felt the full impact of the European invasion. Tribe after tribe of their great Lenape family was wiped out, or reduced to a few remnants. Once-great nations were shattered in the space of a lifetime. Despite all their valor and diplomatic skills, the Lenni Lenape, now called the Delaware Indians, were forced to retreat westward again and again, first to Pennsylvania, then to Ohio, then to Indiana. Through it all, these proud people kept their sense of who they were, and who they had been.

In the summer of 1820, their last villages on the White River in Indiana were being abandoned as the Delawares packed up to leave for new lands west of the Mississippi, where they hoped to be left alone. In one lonely, half-empty village, a deadly epidemic disease struck the family of an Olumpees, a record-keeper. No Indian healer could help him. In despair, the Olumpees turned for help to a white physician named Ward who happened to be passing through, collecting botanical specimens. Dr. Ward succeeded in curing his patient, and the grateful Delaware man gave Dr. Ward his most precious possession: the wooden records containing the symbols of the Red Record. At this moment, the records of the lost age passed from the Indian world to the white world.

Dr. Ward held the wooden records and studied the carefully formed hieroglyphs but could not decipher their meaning. He thought that scholarship could eventually unlock their secret, so he gave the records to his botanist friend Constantine Samuel Rafinesque, a pioneer natural-ist and archeologist who was professor of botany, natural history, and modern languages at Transylvania University in Kentucky, the only university on the frontier. Two years later, in 1822, Rafinesque obtained "from another individual," a transcription of the Delaware lyrics that accompanied the symbols, but because he could find no one to translate these words, he was left as mystified as before. As the historian Paul Weer points out, Rafinesque "was the most qualified individual then in the Ohio Valley to appreciate its value; and yet, in 1824 [when Rafinesque published his *Annals of Kentucky*] he said he had no idea concerning its significance."[5]

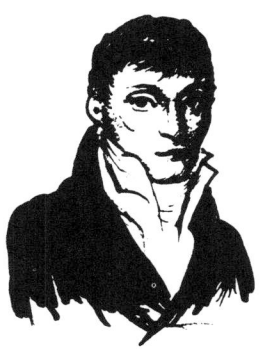

Portrait of Rafinesque. Constantine Rafinesque was the recorder and first translator of the Red Record.

Constantine Rafinesque was a brilliant and prolific, if sometimes eccentric, scientist who laid the groundwork for much of American botany and archeology. One biography says that he "missed greatness by embracing too many fields of knowledge."[6] Yet it was fortunate that he could bring such a wide range of knowledge to the study of the Red Record.

Born in 1787 in Constantinople of French and German-Greek parents and raised in Italy, Rafinesque was a child prodigy, who read a thousand books by the age of twelve and studied fifty different languages by the age of sixteen. In 1802, he made his first trip to the New World, where he met President Jefferson in Washington, D.C., and talked through an interpreter to a delegation of Osage at the Capitol. During this time, he conceived a boundless enthusiasm for the still undescribed natural history of the New World.

After his return to Italy, Rafinesque prospered as a businessman while continuing research into botany and ichthyology. In 1815, he set off for America, laden with specimens and merchandise, only to be washed ashore penniless after a shipwreck that nearly cost him his life. His talents soon enabled him to recover, and through friends he was invited to become a professor at Transylvania University in Kentucky, where he could pursue his travels and collecting throughout the Midwest. He would eventually become the most-traveled American naturalist of his day. When he returned to Philadelphia in 1826, he had a most unusual specimen with him—the Red Record.

Had Rafinesque not been such an eager and avid collector, he might not have taken the time before he left Kentucky to find the words that went with the symbols, and the pictographs would have remained mute forever. And had he not been so free from preconceived ideas about science, willing to examine everything with what a biographer called his "unconquerable innocence," he might never have responded to something as unconventional as the Red Record.[7]

Translating the Past

For the next several years, he traveled and published on many subjects, mostly botany and natural history. With great discipline, he also found the time and energy to undertake, among his many other projects, the translation of the Red Record.

After he returned to Philadelphia, Rafinesque was fortunate to have access to the Moravian Archives nearby in Bethlehem. The Moravians, officially known as the United Brethren, were a Protestant sect who maintained a missionary presence among the Delawares from 1740 to 1808 and who kept voluminous records, including dictionaries and word lists of the Delaware language. Using these, and drawing upon his talents as a linguist, Rafinesque was able to produce a credible, if imperfect, translation despite the unfamiliar language, finally completing this translation in 1833.

He then drew the symbols and wrote the original words and his translation in a couple of small notebooks, which he entitled "Walam Olum: the painted & engraved Traditions of the Linni Lenape" and included the notation that "This Mpt. & the wooden original was procured in 1822 in Kentucky, but was inexplicable until a deep study of the Linapi enabled me to translate them with explanations."[8] He also penciled in "Dr. Ward," apparently to say from whom the materials had come. At the end of the second notebook, Rafinesque also included an English translation of a native Delaware account of their later history that he labeled "Fragment: On the History of the Linapis since abt. 1600, when the Wallamolum closes."

These two notebooks form the Rafinesque Manuscript (see Figure 1.1), the oldest surviving copy of the Red Record and a uniquely valuable document in American history. The only other major clues that Rafi-

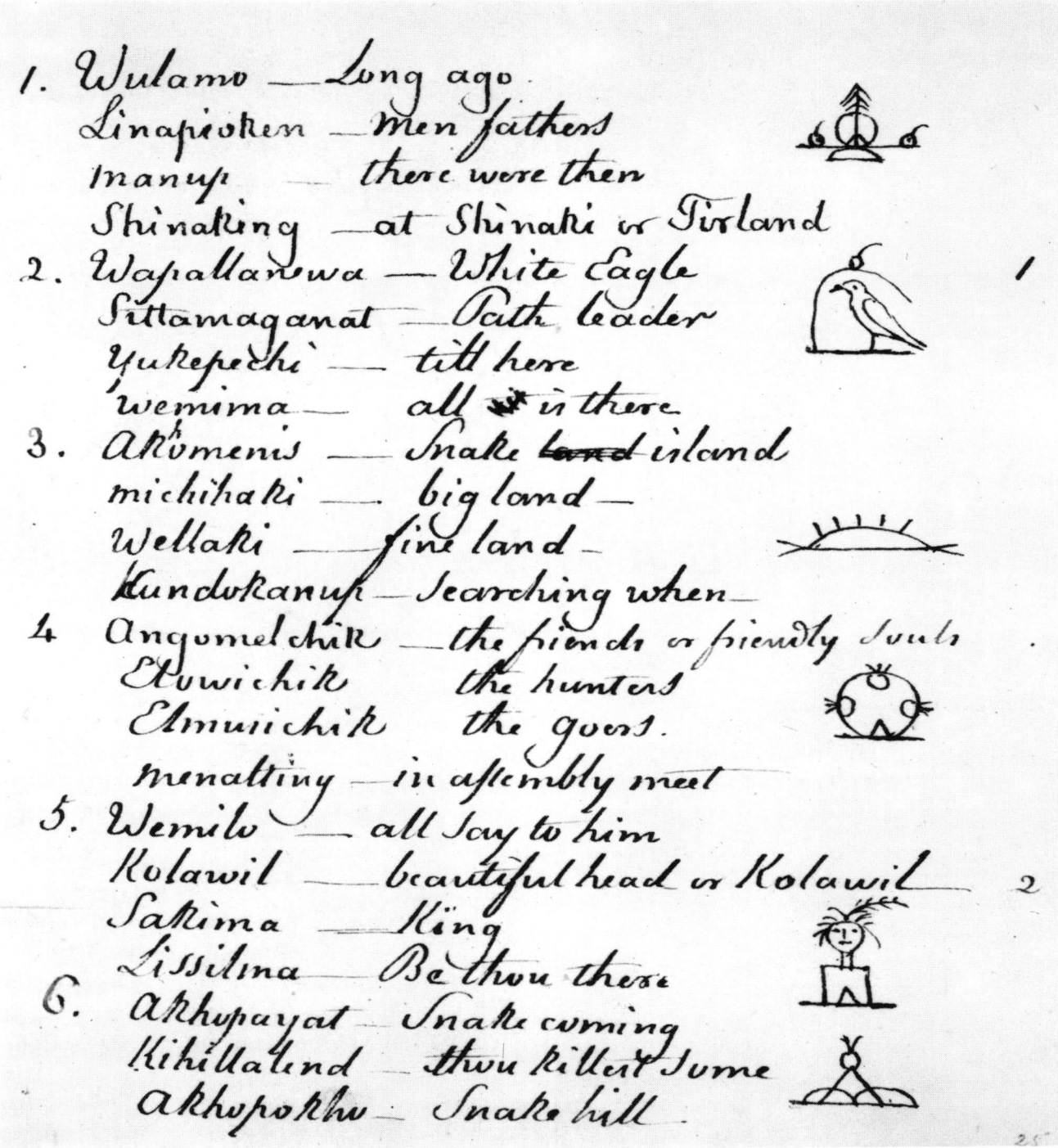

1. Wulamo ― Long ago.
   Linapioken ― Men fathers
   manup ― there were then
   Shinaking ― at Shinaki or Firland
2. Wapallanewa ― White Eagle
   Sittamaganat ― Path leader
   Yukepechi ― till here
   Wemima ― all in there
3. Akomenis ― Snake ~~land~~ island
   michihaki ― big land
   Wellaki ― fine land
   Kundokanup ― Searching when
4. Angomelchik ― the friends or friendly Souls
   Etowichik ― the hunters
   Elmusichik ― the guests.
   menalting ― in assembly meet
5. Wemilo ― all say to him
   Kolawil ― beautiful head or Kolawil
   Sakima ― King
   Lissilma ― Be thou there
6. Akhopayat ― Snake coming
   Kihillalend ― thou killest some
   Akhopokhu ― Snake hill

Figure 1.1. A page from the Rafinesque Manuscript.

nesque left as to the origins of the Red Record are in a book he published at his own expense in 1836 entitled *The American Nations, or Outlines of their General History, Ancient and Modern.* In it, he includes his translation of the Red Record, though without any symbols (possibly because of the cost), and introduces it thus:

> Having obtained through the late Dr. Ward of Indiana, some of the original Wallam-Olum (painted records) of the Linapi tribe of Wapahum or White River, the translation will be given of the songs annexed to each; which form a kind of connected annals of the nation. In the illustrations of this history, will be figured the original glyphs or symbols, and the original songs, with a literal translation word for word. This will furnish a great addition to our knowledge of American graphics and philology; but here the annals are chiefly interesting historically. I have translated, however, all the historical and geographical names, so as to afford [a] better clue to the whole.
>
> We knew by all the writers who had friendly intercourse with the tribes of North America, that they did possess, and perhaps keep yet, historical and traditional records of events, by hieroglyphs or symbols, on wood, bark, skins in stringed wampun, etc.; but none had been published in the original form. This shall be the first attempt.[9]

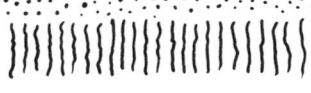

Ojibwa symbol. Chief George Copway's rendering of the Ojibwa symbol for the Grand Medicine Lodge is an example of Ojibwa pictographs.

Rafinesque says "these historical songs of the Linapi, are known to but few individuals, and must be learned with much labor." He goes on to mention several examples of historical records found among Indian tribes, and how "painted tales and annals" could be found among the "Linapi tribes" in particular, from the East Coast to the Midwest.

As to the symbols of the Red Record, Rafinesque says these "when met alone, were inexplicable, but by obtaining the words or verses (since they must commonly be sung) we may acquire enough to lead on further enquiries." He describes how by studying the words of the corresponding verses, the symbols can be seen to contain several combined ideas in compound ideograms. He correctly points out that this makes it different from writing systems such as that of the Maya, which he was among the first to say was partly syllabic. In a perceptive challenge to future scholars, Rafinesque wonders whether a study of these and other Indian writings might lead to the identification of "a peculiar graphic system of North America, different from the Mexican system, and probably once imported from Asia." He points to graphic symbols used by certain Siberian tribes that might provide parallels, symbols that were "indicated by [the distinguished German scholar and explorer] Humboldt but which are unknown to me. Meantime I shall give materials for such researches in my illustrations."

To cover the costs of his scientific work, Rafinesque invented and marketed a vegetable remedy for tuberculosis, and later organized and managed a savings bank, inventing the coupon bond. This talent for business enabled him to publish much that would otherwise have remained unknown, including his first study of the Red Record. A bibliography of his published works contains 938 items. But because he had to work so rapidly, usually without adequate financial support, he sometimes was not able to fully record his facts. What he managed to publish about the Red Record is maddeningly brief, and has been a source of frustration for scholars ever since. The identity of Dr. Ward, for instance, was a mystery until investigation uncovered evidence that the man who first received the Red Record tablets may have been Dr. John Russell Ward, a resident of Carlisle, Kentucky, who died in 1834.[10] Ethnohistory was not really Rafinesque's field of expertise, and he was unaware of how unusual and important the Red Record actually was. His treatment of it seems to have been that of a conscientious amateur, recording and passing on the facts as he knew them in case they would be of interest to other scholars and historians. But the Red Record was ignored.

For the next sixty years, the Red Record was handled with a neglect that seems shocking by modern standards. Perhaps the lack of interest stemmed from an unspoken feeling, even among scholars, that it was better to suppress Indian culture than to preserve it. Several times, the words and symbols of the Red Record came close to being lost forever. The Rafinesque Manuscript, in fact, almost ended up in a garbage heap.

In his last years, Rafinesque worked in increasing isolation. Far ahead of his time in many of his ideas, his genius was wasted on his contemporaries. One reason he never answered the many questions that occur to us now about the origins of the Red Record is that, apparently, no one at the time bothered to ask him. The lack of response to his work led him to a pauper's grave after he died in a garret on September 18, 1840, at the age of fifty-seven. His friends had to smuggle his body out the window to keep his landlord from selling it to a medical school.

Most of his herbarium, reputed to have contained 50,000 specimens collected over a lifetime of travels, was discarded by contemptuous curators. Other men of science got together to save what they could from destruction. An auction of Rafinesque's books and collections brought a total of $131.42. For a few dollars, Professor S.S. Haldeman of the University of Pennsylvania bought the Red Record notebooks and two other manuscripts relating to ancient Indian mounds in Kentucky and neighboring states. After the auction, Rafinesque's unsold specimens and papers, which may have held the answers to our questions, ended up in the Philadelphia public dump.

The Rafinesque Manuscript containing the Red Record next apparently went to a man named Nicollet,[11] and after he died, it came to *Brantz Mayer* of Baltimore, a distinguished amateur antiquarian who had written a best-selling book about the history of Mexico. Mayer was a co-founder of the Maryland Historical Society, and on December 5, 1844, he made a donation to the society's collections. It was recorded thus: "From Brantz Mayer, esq., was received a large collection of rare and curious pamphlets, on various subjects, for the library . . . several autograph letters from persons of distinction; also pieces of birch bark with picture writing and hieroglyphics by northwestern Indians, and other curiousities."[12]

As vague as this is, it does provide an important clue as to what may have happened to the original Red Record pictographs, for in the 1840s "northwestern Indians" referred to those from the old Northwest Territory, which included Indiana. However, there is a very unusual notation next to it: "Withdrawn by him Sept. 29, 1875 B.M." The pictographs have never been heard of since.[13]

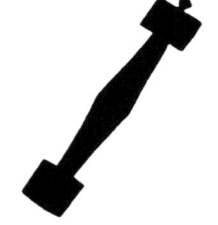

Kickapoo prayer stick. Shown here is an outline of a Kickapoo prayer stick, upon which special symbols would be carved to aid the memory during a prayer or recitation.

These symbols may have come to Rafinesque on pieces of birch bark or wood, or possibly a combination of both. He was unclear on this point, but did mention "wooden originals" on which the symbols were "painted & engraved." Let us hope that they have not been lost forever. The historical importance of these fragile wooden documents is by now almost incalculable.

Scholars Take a Second Look

In 1846, Mayer loaned the Rafinesque Manuscript and some of his other papers to the pioneer American archeologist Ephraim G. Squier, who was then writing, with E.H. Davis, the classic *Ancient Monuments of the Mississippi Valley* for the fledgling Smithsonian Institution. Squier made use of Rafinesque's studies of ancient earthworks in the Ohio valley, and became increasingly interested in the Red Record. He based his studies on the manuscript alone, for there is no evidence that he ever saw the original carved pictographs. In 1848, Squier wrote a paper entitled "Historical and Mythological Traditions of the Algonquins; with a Translation of the Walum-Olum, or Bark Record of the Lenni-Lenape," which was read before a meeting of the New York Historical Society and later published. In the paper, he expressed his conviction that the Wallam Olum was what it seemed to be—a genuine Indian record, and not a forgery. Furthermore, his native informant, George Copway, the distinguished Ojibwa chief, unhesitatingly pronounced the story to be consistent with other known Algonquian religious and historical traditions.[14]

Squier felt the Red Record was worthy of serious attention. But for the next thirty-five years, as Native American nations in the West continued to be destroyed, the Red Record was ignored. Perhaps this was because Squier's translation, which was a paraphrase of Rafinesque's, was still disjointed and hard to follow. A new attempt was needed to bring the Lenni Lenape and their history into perspective.

The noted scholar Dr. Daniel G. Brinton, in his 1883 book *Aboriginal American Authors*, was the next to mention the Red Record. He managed to trace the Rafinesque Manuscript to Squier, but concluded by saying, "I have been unable to find the original."

Soon afterward, however, he was able to recover the manuscript, if not the original wooden records, from the family of the late Brantz Mayer, and he made it the subject of a major study, published in 1884, entitled *The Lenâpé and their Legends: with the Complete Text and Symbols of the Walam Olum, a New Translation, and an Inquiry into its Authenticity.* This was the first major examination of the context as well as the content of the Red Record, and it contains much valuable background information, as well as an improved translation and the first publication of the symbols. Then Brinton donated the Rafinesque Manuscript to the University of Pennsylvania at Philadelphia, where today it can be found in the Van Pelt-Dietrich Library Center, Department of Special Collections, in the heart of what was once the homeland of the Lenni Lenape.

Despite Brinton's work, the Red Record was still being ignored eight years after his publication. In the frenzy of celebrations marking the 400th anniversary of the "Discovery of America" in 1892, the official line was that American history began with Columbus, and this fiction continued to fill the textbooks. It was more convenient for Americans to believe that this continent was empty before the colonists came, or, at most, inhabited by people incompetent to record their past history.

As the twentieth century began, the remaining Delawares struggled to overcome the general indifference to Native American culture. Richard G. Adams, a Delaware attorney, managed to publish, at his own expense, a series of illustrated books recording the legends and traditions of his people. From the 1920s through the 1940s, pioneering anthropologists such as Mark Harrington and Frank G. Speck recorded glimpses of vanishing Delaware customs and traditions from among the last survivors in Oklahoma and Canada. But the most complete and challenging legacy of the Lenni Lenape, the Red Record, still awaited full examination and explanation.

Finally, in 1954, the Indiana Historical Society published a handsome volume entitled *Walam Olum or Red Score: The Migration Legend of the Lenni Lenape or Delaware Indians, a New Translation, Interpreted by Linguistic, Historical, Archeological, Ethnological, and Physical Anthropological Studies.*

This book contained the results of a comprehensive twenty-year study of the background and meaning of the Rafinesque Manuscript and its contents. It also included a facsimile reproduction of the manuscript itself, so that the original words, which had too often been misspelled in past studies, and the symbols, which had been badly drawn, distorted, omitted, or even reproduced upside down, could be seen clearly at last. In addition, the book contained valuable research on the background, history, and meaning of the Red Record. It concluded, like Squier, Brinton, Speck, Harrington, and their native informants had concluded in the past, that the Red Record was created by the Delawares, and was representative of their known historical and religious traditions. However, the featured new translation, by focusing on secondary meanings in the words and neglecting readability and logical sense in English, was harder to follow than ever.

Bringing the Picture Into Focus

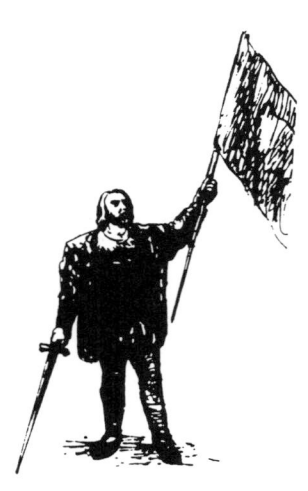

So the Red Record remained relatively unknown to the general public. Poor translations and the loss of the original tablets have done much to keep the Red Record from being widely known. But ignorance, prejudice, and fear may also have played a part. Americans' ignorance of the traditions and culture that preceded them and produced the Red Record may have been "blissful," preventing feelings of guilt and permitting a sense of superiority. Guilt feelings were also held at bay by the preconceived notion that any form of oral tradition was historically useless, and that Native Americans were not capable of maintaining a written history of ancient times. But white Americans have not been alone in their resistance to the Red Record.

The description in the Red Record of a crossing of the Bering Strait raises understandable concerns among contemporary Native Americans. Too often, talk of a migration from Asia to America has been used to imply that Native Americans are immigrants just like everyone else, and thus have no aboriginal rights. But Native Americans have been on this continent more than 36,000 years.[15] It is presumptuous to equate the European experience of America, only a small fraction of this length of time, to the Native Americans' experience, which is so strongly characterized by the deepest reverence for and attachment to this land of their birth.

Furthermore, the description in the Red Record of the Lenape crossing the Bering Strait into America never says that they were the first or only ones to do so. The Red Record clearly states that when the Lenape crossed into America it was *already* inhabited, and many comments are made

Conventional image of Columbus, here depicted as "The Discoverer."

about the other tribes that the Lenape encountered on their journey across the continent. Although ancestors of Native Americans did indeed cross into this continent, this event has too often been misinterpreted. Actually, it only tells half of the story. The Bering Strait throughout much of its history was a land bridge, and, like any bridge, it could be used for travel in *both* directions. It is even possible that the ancestors of the Lenape originated in America, and that Book II of the Red Record is a symbolic story of their first crossing—into Asia.

To better understand the Red Record, we must have a clear picture of what it is and what it says. This edition contains the clearest presentation yet of the symbols, text, and probable meaning of the Red Record. With this information, we can begin the process of examination that will help the Red Record emerge from obscurity to become a well-known part of our national heritage.

The Red Record can extend the American heritage back into the far distant past. It speaks of times long, long ago, as far back as—or farther than—the earliest Maya records, which date from around 312 A.D.[16] Does this mean that the Red Record itself is almost 1,500 years old? Although it draws from a much older body of traditions, the Red Record itself is first mentioned in the summer of 1820, when its symbols were given to Dr. Ward. The Moravian missionaries, who lived among the Lenni Lenape until 1806, did not describe it. But this is probably because it was kept by a select few elders who were trained as historians, and only brought out and sung on special occasions, such as the annual sacred Big House Ceremony, which the missionaries and other whites were not allowed to attend. Many aspects of Delaware culture were understandably kept secret from a white culture that too often ridiculed and tried to suppress Native American culture. It was not until well into the twentieth century that the Delawares were allowed to practice their ancient religion legally and openly. Perhaps this prejudice is another reason why acceptance of the historical traditions embodied in the Red Record has been so long in coming.

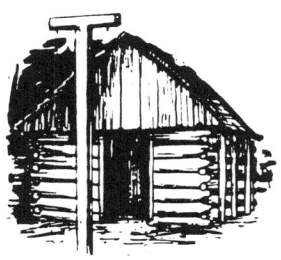

Entrance to Big House. The last big house was located near Copan, Oklahoma.

One theory about the age of the Red Record was advanced by the anthropologist William Newcomb. He suggested that the Red Record was composed shortly before 1820, during the religious and cultural revival movement centered around Tecumseh and his twin brother Tenskwatawa, the Shawnee Prophet, in an effort to revive the failing traditions and prestige of the Delawares. Because the Delawares at the time were so disorganized and demoralized, Newcomb says, such a story would be a product of wishful thinking rather than historical facts—"an account . . . of a Golden Age which never was."[17]

This is a denial of the capacity of any Native Americans to record history. Even if the Red Record were composed shortly before 1820, leaving aside the many indications within it of a much greater age, it more likely would have been a sincere attempt by one or more Delawares to record what were believed to be the facts of their history before they were lost forever. If a great catastrophe had destroyed all historical records and a group of well-read, educated Americans were asked to write a brief summation of Western history, including the ancient world, Medieval Europe, and the exploration and colonization of the Americas, the resulting synthesis of remembered history might contain some mistakes, but it would undoubtedly be an honest effort to preserve the bare facts for future generations. The original occupants of America would undoubtedly do no less to preserve the essentials of that age when America was theirs alone.

The Red Record is a remarkable story indeed. It is a song of great beginnings, of travels on foot across vast landscapes fresh from the hand of the Creator. Here are hints of once-famous personalities: the visionary Wapallanewa, the White Eagle, who first led the way to the New World; the ruthless Ayamek, the Seizer; the embattled Opekasit; the traveling prophet Onowutok; the great Tamanend the First; and the treacherous King of the Talegas. There is even a glimpse of the ancient historians Olumapi and Lekhihiten, recording the memories of the past. We catch the last echoes of the once-mighty names and deeds of the First Age, reverberating down through the centuries. Now our imaginations, as well as our scholarship, are needed to bring this story back to life.

The story told in the Red Record is Chapter One of the story of America. It is the only written link to our uttermost past.

Chapter Two

Unlocking the Story

The Red Record is a fascinating mystery, full of secrets. Past attempts at translation have failed to reveal all it contains and have fallen into muddled language and confusing interpretations. But by long, careful and systematic examination of the evidence, a clearer picture emerges, one that includes unsuspected depth and dimension. Although the Red Record is brief, its words and symbols can be seen to contain a wealth of information; in addition to its uniquely valuable account of past events, it includes a time scale covering more than a thousand years, and an accurate record of travel over thousands of miles, following a migration route that stretches back into Asia.

The language and form of the Red Record are distinctive. Its 687 words are the lyrics of a song, cryptic, poetic, highly compressed. It is in an archaic form of the language, like the English of Shakespeare or the King James Bible.[1] One reason the Red Record has been so difficult to translate until now is the density of meaning packed into each of its carefully chosen words. These describe the essence of events, citing only the most important details. But these words probably were intended to remind the original audience of other, more complete accounts they had heard elsewhere, stories that have now almost all been lost. It is like an old painting whose colors have grown dim but whose outlines remain clear.

The compressed, evocative nature of the words of the Red Record is consistent with descriptions of the Lenape language. William Penn, for example, called the language "lofty, yet narrow, but like the Hebrew; in Signification full, like short-hand in writing; one word serveth the place of three, and the rest are supplied by the Understanding of the Hearer . . . And I must say, that I know not a Language spoken in Europe, that hath words of more sweetness or greatness, in Accent and Emphasis, than theirs."[2]

Previous translations of the Red Record have tended to be contradictory and hard to follow. The best sources for determining the most accurate translation of the words are the word lists written by the Moravian missionaries who lived among the Delawares from 1755 until 1808. These word lists reflect the Delaware language as it was spoken at the time the Red Record was recorded by Rafinesque. The most complete of these word lists, A *Lenâpé-English Dictionary,* was published in 1888 by Daniel G. Brinton with annotations by the Reverend A.S. Anthony, a Delaware familiar with the language as it was then spoken among the Delaware survivors in Canada. More recent descriptions of the language— such as those by Nora Thompson Dean, one of the last fluent Delaware speakers in Oklahoma—and contemporary academic studies by Carl Vogelin, Jim Rementer, and Jay Miller have also added to our understanding of the words of the Red Record. A guide to the pronunciation of these words was left by Rafinesque: "The orthography of the Linapi names is reduced to the Spanish and French pronunciation, except for *sh* as in English, *u* as in French, *w* as *hou.*"[3]

The 183 symbols of the Red Record are as important as the words in many ways. As a mnemonic aid, they originally helped the singer recall the words and the order of events. Now they help the translator as well, by showing which meaning or nuance of the words is intended. They are very evocative and follow a consistent system for expressing meaning in abstract symbols—an evolving form of writing in ideograms. A listing of the apparent meanings of some basic symbols appears in Table 2.1. Combinations of these basic forms are used to represent complex combinations of ideas.

These symbols mirror examples of pictographic records found among other Lenape tribes. Several of the symbols in the Red Record's earliest sections also bear a remarkable resemblance, both in form and in meaning, to the oldest forms of writing in ancient China, and hint at profound antiquity.[4]

As the meanings of symbols and words emerge, it becomes obvious that they contain many references to ancient Lenni Lenape legends and

Table 2.1. Selected symbols used by the Lenni Lenape or Delaware Indians in their historical and religious testament, the Wallam Olum or Red Record.

Symbol	Meaning	Symbol	Meaning
○	–Spirited, living thing	—	–Ground level
⊙	–Spirit or manito	=	–Earth
◇⊙	–Great Spirit	≡	–Homeland
⌒	–Island, land	⌣	–Body of water
△	–Cold	☀	–Rising Sun
△	–Fire (council fire)	□	–An establishment
△	–Capital	⊓	–Town
⧻	–Difficulty, danger	≢	–Prosperity
♀	–Ancient Lenape (Algonquian) person	✕	–War
♀	–Modern Lenape chief	♀	–Holy man
♀	–Lenape person	♀	–Strong chief
♀	–Snake (enemy)	♀	–Iroquois
♂	–Talega (Moundbuilder)	♀	–White person

traditions. Understanding the references requires a knowledge of Lenape practices. Fortunately, many of the Lenni Lenape traditions were recorded at an early date because the Lenni Lenape were among the first tribes with whom the Europeans had contact in what is now the United States. Additional information on the meaning of these references may be gleaned from the Lenni Lenape's widespread Lenape tribal relatives, many of whom survived—along with their traditions—in a more intact condition than did the Delawares. By a wide search of the legends and traditions of both the Delawares and their Lenape family relations, it is possible to find parallel accounts of and explanations for many of the incidents in the story.

Anthropology and archeology are also of great help in piecing together what may have happened. The Red Record describes events in many regions of North America; the Lenape or Algonquian language group was the most widespread native language group on the continent. Many Lenape tribes were later encountered living in the places featured in the story, and serve as examples of Lenni Lenape life in those regions in the distant past. Even in places outside of the later range of the Lenape, such as Alaska and the Northwest Coast, other indigenous tribes indicate what life may have been like for the Lenape when they lived there.

By applying all of this evidence, we arrive at a clearer picture of the meaning of the symbols and words. We come to a better understanding of who did what, and of why it was done. But the Red Record also contains clues that enable us to learn *when* events may have taken place.

A time scale for the Red Record is easily established; the greater part of the account, Books IV and V, includes a listing of ninety-six successive national leaders, so events are dateable according to the number of the reigning leader. Though this approach is approximate, it can serve as a basis for chronology. But it remains an open question whether the mention of a leader represents the span of time of a generation, or only of the years of the leader's reign. Also, although the leaders listed probably follow each other in order, at least some could have been contemporaries, such as those whose symbols are shown side by side. Reigns must have had different lengths, but a sense of the average can be determined based on the average length of the reigns during the period where dates can be established using a method first described by the industrialist and antiquarian Eli Lilly in the 1954 Indiana Historical Society study of the Red Record.[5]

As Lilly pointed out, the earliest dateable event in the Red Record is suggested by a calendar belt of black wampum beads counting the years since the arrival of the Lenni Lenape on the East Coast at the conclusion of their migration, as noted in the Red Record (V:26). When counted in 1766, this calendar belt revealed that the date of the arrival was 1396.[6]

The Red Record also notes the first arrival of European explorers (V:40), probably referring to Verrazano's visit in 1524, and later ends with the landing of the first European colonists around 1620 (V:60). After this, a historical "Fragment" at the end of the Rafinesque Manuscript (see page 148) lists the Delaware chiefs from 1620 up until 1820. From 1396 to the end of the Fragment in 1820 is a span of 424 years in which a total of 31 chiefs is mentioned in the Red Record and the Fragment. The average reign is, therefore, approximately 13.67 years. Lilly points out that this is comparable to the fifteen-year average of other dynasties such as the Sumerians, the Aztecs, and the ancient Hawaiians. So as an approximation, a rough date for an event can be calculated according to the number of the reign or generation named. Since Books IV and V cover 96 generations, the story therein spans 1,312 years, beginning in 308 A.D., the same time as the start of Mayan records, and ending in 1620. If the average reign is actually longer than fifteen years, or if some chiefs have been omitted, then the starting date is even earlier. Rafinesque, for instance, assumed that each reign represented a generation of around 33 years, which placed the starting date at 1600 B.C.

We will probably never know for certain when the Red Record was composed, but the last verse is an important indicator of its antiquity: "Friendly people, in great ships; who are they?" (V:60). The Lenni Lenape quickly found out who the Europeans were, to their regret. But no trace of this disturbs the innocence of this last verse. So it, like the rest of the verses, seems to be preserved from pre-colonial times.

Establishing locations for the events in the Red Record is even easier than establishing dates, but requires a different kind of analysis. Eli Lilly was also the first to theorize that the Red Record can be understood as a record of a journey eastward out of Asia across North America (see Figure 2.1 on pages 20 and 21), with clues in the words and symbols that point to specific locations along the way. To test this theory, maps of the actual landscape were compared to the descriptions of the journey. This analysis, detailed in the Appendix (page 183), reveals not only the startling accuracy of the Red Record's description of the migration route shown in Figure 2.1, but also important clues as to how, when, and why the Red Record was composed.

Retracing the Journey

The words and symbols of the Red Record indicate many features of the landscape that were noted by the Lenape during the journey. Oceans, shorelines, forests, grasslands, and prevailing climates are mentioned, and there are lakes, rivers, and even waterfalls that are specifically named.

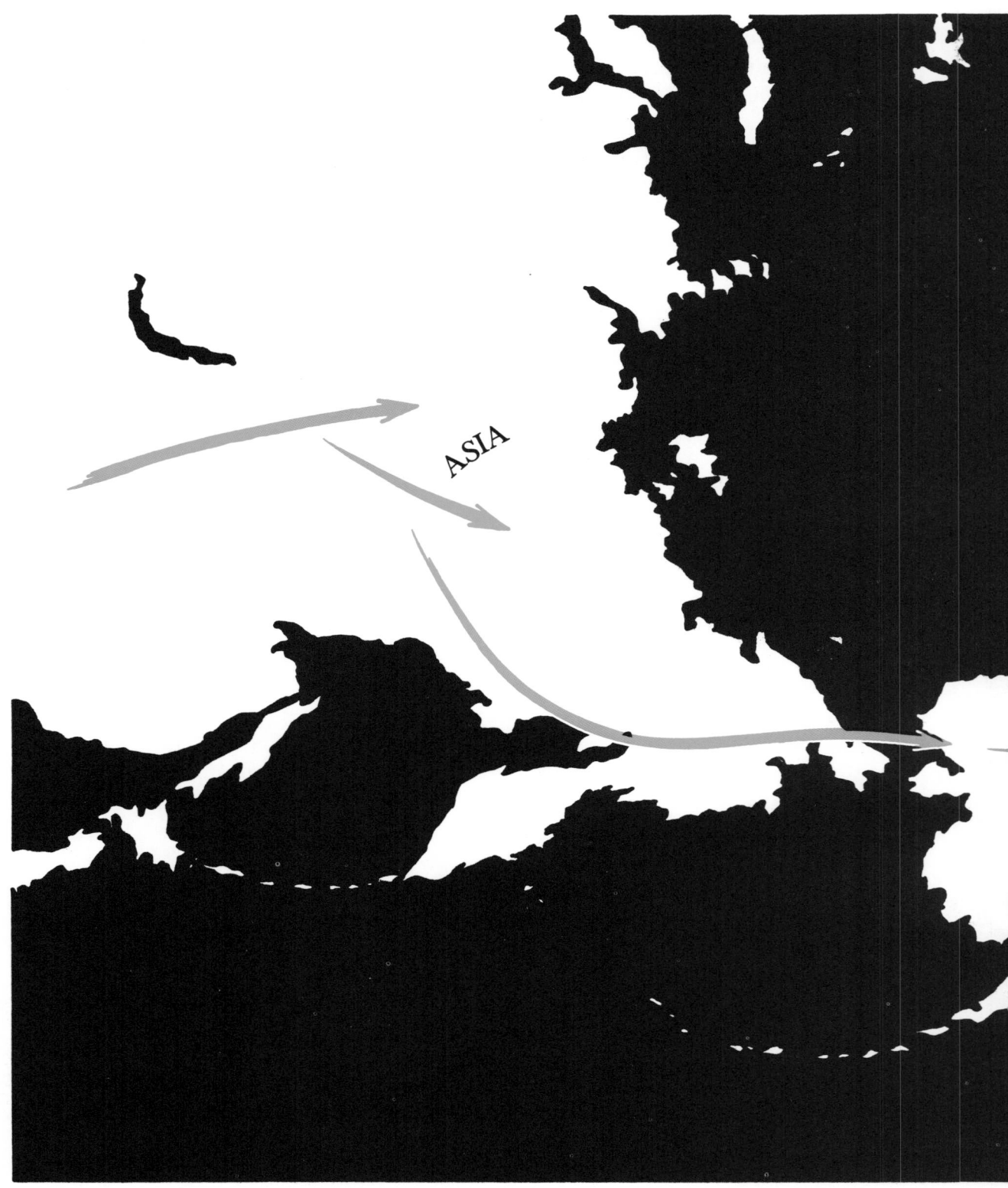

Figure 2.1. The migration route of the Lenni Lenape. The arrows depict the path of the Lenni Lenape as they journeyed out of Asia to the North Ameri-

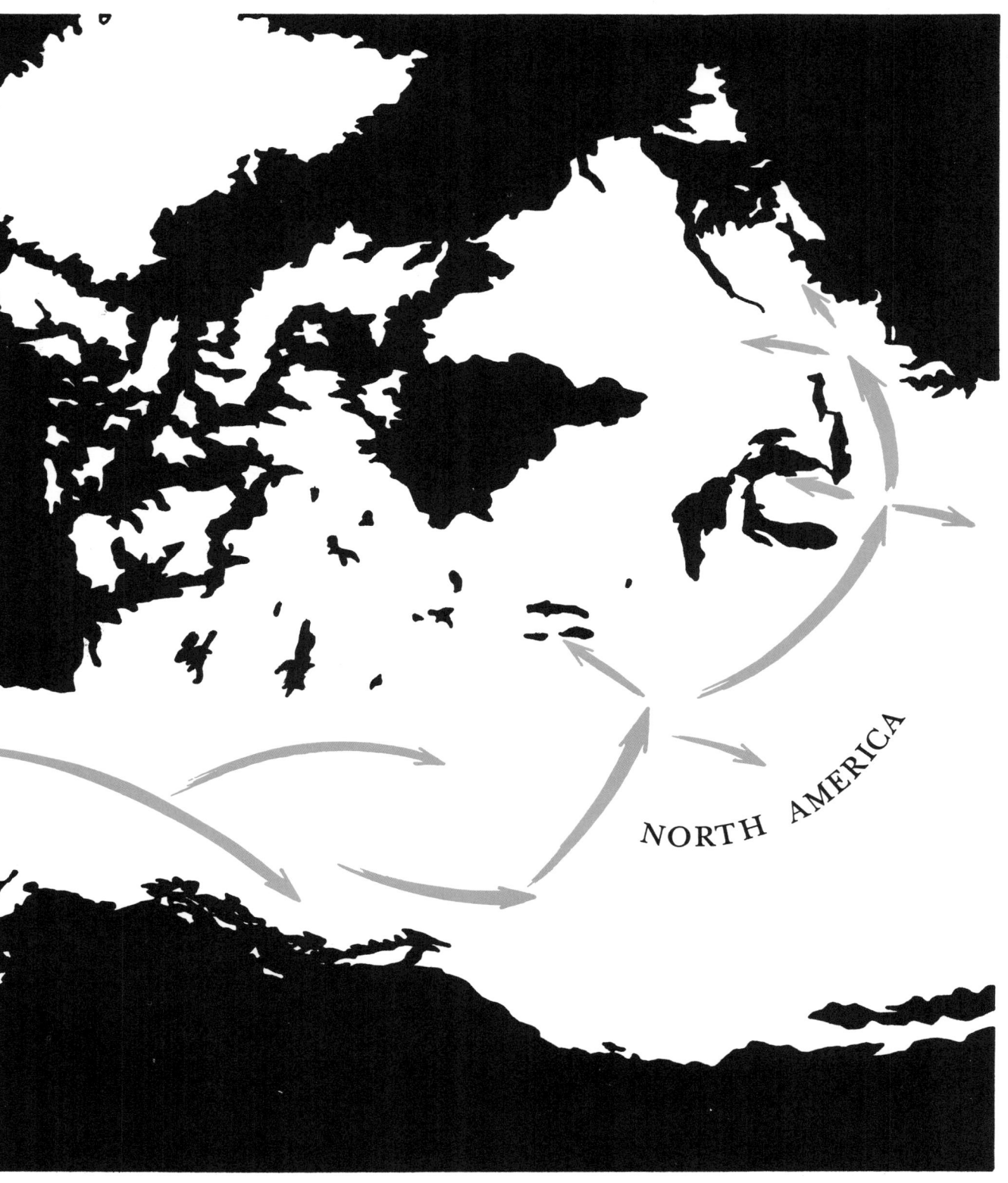

can continent. The migration route depicted here is based upon the text of
the Red Record as well as on the author's research.

By following the trail backward, recognizing and identifying the landscape features as they appear, we can retrace the epic journey back to its beginning in the most distant past.

We know that when the European colonists came, the Lenni Lenape were living along the East Coast, centered in the Delaware valley. The identities of the geographical locations mentioned at the end of Book V are therefore obvious, especially as several of these features still bear remnants of the original Indian names mentioned in the text, such as the Allegheny Mountains and the Susquehanna River. We also can identify the symbols for the Mississippi River and the White River in Indiana both because of their mention in the words and the strong Delaware traditions concerning both places.

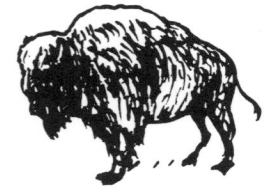

Buffalo.
Millions of buffalo once roamed the Great Plains.

Other landscape features further westward are indicated in the Red Record: a great range of mountains like the Rockies, and a fruitful river identified as the "Yellow River" (IV:34), which could be the Yellowstone. In addition, there are descriptions of herds of buffalo, which are a well-known feature of the aboriginal Great Plains. A count of the generations in the Red Record, using a conservative figure of 13.67 years each, indicates that the Lenape first crossed the Rockies into the High Plains around 808 A.D.

West of the Rockies, an earlier way of life centered on gathering rather than hunting is described in the Red Record, a way of life characteristic of the Great Plateau and the land to the south in the Great Basin. Here the Lenape are described as raising crops of corn for the first time, after having come south from a much colder region. The changes described in the Red Record match the climatic differences between the Great Plateau and the Canadian Rockies to the north, and the difference in the foods found in each place.

Following the story back in time, we continue to find correspondences between the landscape features mentioned in the Red Record and the landscape features still found on the map today: the "tall pine country, seashore country" (IV:13) matches the region today called the Northwest Coast; the "fishing country, mountain country, game herd country" (IV:14) matches the Yukon and Northwest territories. The Red Record describes this period as a confusing time. The tribe had divided earlier, around 380 A.D. according to a count of the generations; some had gone south along the shore and some had continued east into the hunting country inland. There was a time of great violence and confusion, and apparently the Lenape were in danger of losing their cohesiveness and their historical memory, until Olumapi, History Man (IV:23) appeared. He is given credit for the invention of the first written records.

Symbol for Olumapi.
This symbol for Olumapi, originator of written records, comes from the Red Record.

Other landmarks appear further to the west, landmarks encountered even earlier in time. Before the tribal division, the Lenape are described as living in a wooded vale to the northwest that matches the characteristics of the Yukon River valley in Alaska. Studies have shown that the Yukon valley remained a relatively green and ice-free haven even around the time of the Ice Age.

The Red Record describes a wide ice-covered strait west of this green refuge, over which the Lenape crossed to begin a new life. Surprising as this may seem, logic and the abundance of specific description in the symbols and the words lead to the conclusion that this landscape feature is the Bering Strait, and that the crossing described in the Red Record is a migration from Asia to America.

The Bering Strait is described in unusual detail in the story, which concurs with its importance in the Lenape saga. It is described more completely than any other landscape feature in the Red Record. Because of the size of this land bridge, its crossing occupies the entire last half of Book III, and the completion of this crossing literally begins a new chapter—Book IV—in the Lenape history.

The words emphasize that the crossing was a fundamental change. The Red Record mentions that the northeastern clans initiated the migration, which was undertaken with great reluctance by the western clans who preferred to remain where they were. Apparently this was a crossing that was not easily accomplished, and there was no turning back. The extent of the description of the reason, method, participants and time involved in the crossing shows that it was a much more formidable task than the crossing of a river. A river crossing is only mentioned once, in passing, when the Lenape cross the great Mississippi.

There are also unusually detailed descriptions of the Bering Strait and the way it was crossed, and the details are all remarkably consistent with the actual characteristics of this area both today and in the past. The area is described as "the dark fish sea, the gaping hollow sea" (III,12), which may refer to the overcast skies, rich marine life, and strong tides characteristic of the Bering Sea. After the Ice Age, when the sea level was lower than it is today, the Bering Strait would have been a foggy channel swept by strong tides, where migrating whales swam between the Arctic and the Pacific oceans.

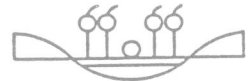

Symbol for the Bering Strait. A crossing of the Bering Strait is apparently depicted in this symbol from the Red Record.

The first crossings by the Lenape are described as being accomplished by rowing, perhaps during the summer, when it was discovered that the land to the east was better than the land to the west. This is true today of the difference between eastern Siberia and Alaska, and it was also true in the past. The actual crossing of the "icy ocean" (III,16) is described in unusual detail: "On a wondrous sheet of ice, all crossed the frozen sea, at low tide in the narrows of the ocean" (III,17). The crossing is described as happening "in a night," which may mean in the dark of an Arctic winter. Because there is snow for the runners of sleds, winter is the time for long journeys in the Arctic, and the most likely time for the Strait to freeze over, as it occasionally does today.

The Bering Strait may be represented in the symbols as many as seven times. Since a semicircle is the symbol of a continent or large island—such as "Turtle Island," the aboriginal name for North America—showing the strait as a passage between two semicircles is a way of showing that it was a passage from one continent to another.

The weight of so many consistent details and descriptions leads one to the conclusion that the landscape feature being crossed here is the Bering Strait and no other. With the Bering Strait thus established as a landmark, following the trail back from there into Asia will enable us to see if the landscape features described in the Red Record continue to match the features on the map. If they do, then the historical accuracy of the Red Record, even at such a great remove of space and time, is maintained, and we have an idea of the starting point of the migration.

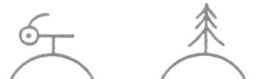

Symbol for two continents. This symbol from the Red Record includes indications of two continents, one on either side of the Bering Strait.

Finding the Starting Point

To retrace the Lenape journey in Book III, we must go deep into the most distant regions and the most distant historical past described in the Red Record. Here there is no chronicle of successive chiefs to supply a measure of time. Here there are indications of movement and landscape, but time is compressed, approaching the mythic dimension found in Book II, the Deluge, and Book I, the Creation. To understand the earliest stage of the journey represented in Book III, we must learn about the topography of the land of Asia.

Eastern Siberia is a vast country, as large as the United States. To the north, the North Slope's cold dry tundra extends eastward in a long peninsula of barren mountains leading to the Bering Strait. In the center, beyond low ranges of windswept mountains, are the evergreen taiga forests of the vast plain watered by the great Lena River, a river longer than the Mississippi. In the south, the Stanovoi and Yablonovyy mountain barriers rise; hidden between them to the west lies the mysterious immensity of Lake Baikal—"Lake of the Spirits"—the deepest lake in the world. Farther south, beyond Siberia, lie the Great Khingan Mountains, between the Gobi Desert and the fertile plains of China.

Any journey northeastward from the vicinity of China to the Bering Strait would encompass five types of climate and terrain on the way: first, the mountains of the Great Khingan barrier and the rolling Yablonovoyy and Stanovoi ranges north of them; second, the plains and rivers of the Lena River basin; third, the frozen tundra of the North Slope; fourth, the barren mountains of the Chukchi Peninsula; fifth, the seashore of the Sea of Okhotsk and the Bering Sea. So the sequence can be described as: mountains—river plain—tundra—barrens—seashore. This sequence mirrors the descriptions of the landscape in the Red Record.

The evidence in the words and symbols of Book III clearly indicates how, from the cold mountains of their first home, the Lenape hunters followed the herds and the rivers northward, spreading into the snowy tundra of the North Slope. When their enemies fled eastward across the rugged and barren wastelands, the Lenape pursued them until they reached the shore, from which Lenape explorers rowing eastward discovered America.

The sequence of landscape features in the Red Record is consistent with a journey out of Asia and across North America. But the Red Record contains even more than just the listing of these features; it also contains an accurate measurement of the distances between them, expressed as increments of movement—steps to the north, south, east, or west—noted in either the symbols or the words.

With a basic scale of roughly 216 miles per step, there is an almost perfect match between the described journey and the actual landscape, with very few adjustments required, all the way from the area of Manchuria to the area of Idaho. Then, from Idaho to Missouri, the scale can be seen to diminish to three-quarters of the original distance per step, then one-half per step from Missouri to West Virginia, and finally to one-third per step from West Virginia to the East Coast and the end of the journey. (For more details, see Appendix.) This gradually diminishing scale is evidence of the length of time over which the Red Record was accumulated, because earlier movements would tend to be remembered with less resolution and detail than more recent ones.

The discovery that the Red Record contains an accurate, systematic geographic record, according to a gradually diminishing scale of distance as events approach the present, gives us insight into how and when the Red Record was composed; it shows that it was the result of a very disciplined, rigorous, long-term effort by the Lenape to ensure the preservation of their story.

There are many clues that the Red Record preserves a firsthand experience of a long-ago crossing of this continent. The completeness and logic of the narrative of the epic journey, and the accuracy of the details noted along the way, including details of distant wildlife and arctic landscapes that a lone Native American author in Indiana would be unlikely to know, argue that these details and events had been preserved from an earlier time, and passed on verbatim in the chronicle even if their meaning was not fully understood. The accuracy of distances and landmarks, even in distant regions, suggests that the Red Record was the result of a long, careful, and extremely

Symbol for the Ice Age. A very early time of great cold is represented by this symbol from the Red Record.

conservative process of composition, based on direct accumulated experience preserved over a long span of time.

During a long migration, people would be able to accurately describe the lay of the land in their immediate vicinity, but as time passed and their migration continued, there would come a time when they would be too far away to revisit regions they had inhabited long before. The span of years as much as the span of distance would threaten their memory, putting the deeds and even the names of their ancestors in danger of being forgotten.

Purely oral traditions tend to break down over long periods of time. As generations go by, the vagaries of memory begin to add up and facts begin to disappear. Yet by a systematic effort of memory, assisted by written symbols, the essentials of history can be preserved, despite the passing generations. In fact, this is what seems to have taken place in the Red Record. First, after twenty-four generations had passed since the crossing of the Bering Strait (taking each described change in national leadership as a generation), there is Olumapi, History Man, who is credited with the beginning of written records. Then, thirty-six generations later, there is Lekhihiten, the Author, recording the Wallam Olum or Red Record. (Unwritten traditions are often given a limit of 500 years before they become inaccurate; if these thirty-six generations represent a 500-year span, this would be 13.88 years per generation, almost exactly the same as the previously estimated 13.67 years per reign.) Another thirty-six generations are described before the Red Record ends.

Over such a span of time, ninety-six generations, one would expect the tale to become more systematic and schematized. This is common among oral traditions because a formalized structure such as a song aids memorization. To enable the tale to be recited in one performance, it would also have to be compressed. The challenge would be to preserve the essentials of the story, in the proper balance, during this process of reduction and crystallization. That this was apparently done successfully can be shown in the accuracy with which the journey is described. This accuracy implies that at least some of the names and deeds described may be accurate as well. The artistic power of the symbols is also evidence of much care and skill.

There is a progressive stylistic simplification of both the words and the symbols as the story moves from ancient toward modern times, showing a process of evolution in both the words and the symbols. The most picture-like symbols are in the early sections, with almost proselike descriptions, while the later parts have streamlined, abstract symbols and very few words—four per verse in Book IV, and only three per verse in Book V. These stylistic changes also suggest that the story may have had more than one author; the account does imply that Lekhihiten, the Author (V:5), may have written Book IV, while Olumapi, History Man

Symbol for Lekhihiten. The symbol of Lekhihiten, an author of the Red Record, is included in that account.

(IV:23), may have helped preserve the earlier sections.

If the account were told and retold over a long span of time, the people and events would become as they are here, reduced to their essential details, mere ciphers to remind the singer and the audience of more complete tales of each period. To sing such a long history with more detail would have taken an inordinate length of time, and been too difficult to remember and teach accurately. So the Red Record may have been intended as a kind of textbook, a codified "pocket history" of the nation for the benefit of the young, to keep them acquainted with the outlines of their heritage.

Through the words and symbols of the Red Record, we find guides to an exploration of the New World that predates Columbus by almost 1,000 years. Knowledge of the ancient traditions—the times, places, people, and events—of the Lenni Lenape can help us to "discover" America at the dawn of its history.

Chapter Three

The Traditions of the Lenni Lenape

The United States is not the first nation to occupy its part of North America, nor is it likely to be the last. Like clouds across the land, successive groups have swept across the continent in the thousands of years of its human habitation. The most recent wave of migration was westward, establishing the territories of the United States. But in the shadowy age before the coming of the European colonists, other nations arose and fell, nations made up of the groups now called the Indian tribes. These tribal nations included absolute monarchies and loose confederations, elective republics, and hereditary plutocracies. But all shared a sense of concern for the welfare of the land. Even after thousands of years of Indian occupation, the land seemed to the Europeans to be essentially untouched, and several explorers likened its beauty to Paradise.

Five hundred years ago, the area of North America that is now the northeastern United States would have appeared from the air as an almost unbroken sea of trees. This great primordial forest was dominated by massive evergreens and deciduous hardwoods in groves so dense that sometimes the shade beneath them was as dark as night. A squirrel could jump from limb to limb from the East Coast almost to the Mississippi.

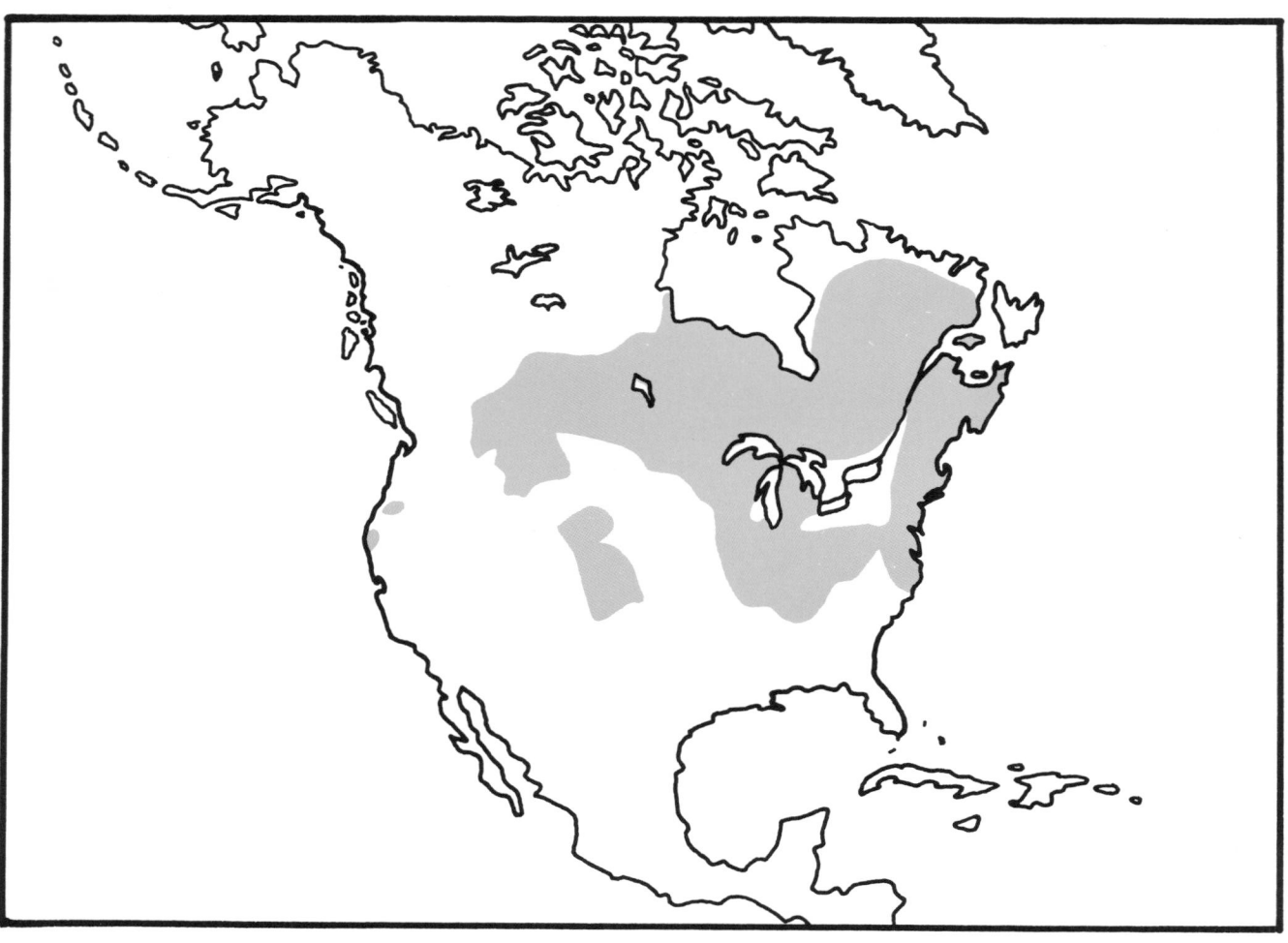

Figure 3.1. Shaded areas show the greatest recorded extent of Algonquian-speaking tribes through the seventeenth, eighteenth, and nineteenth centuries.

This forest area, from beyond the St. Lawrence and the Great Lakes in the north to the Ohio Valley in the south, and from the Atlantic Coast in the east to the Mississippi in the west, formed a region called the Eastern Woodlands.

Within the Eastern Woodlands, rivers and streams wound like silver threads. Along them, one might occasionally glimpse the clearings and villages of the human inhabitants. These forest people mostly belonged to one of two distinct language groups: the Algonquian-speaking tribes (see Figure 3.1), and the Iroquoian-speaking tribes, with the Iroquoians' territory forming an island in the midst of the larger area of the Algonquian-speaking tribes. This Iroquoian island stretched from the populous Wyandots on the Great Lakes in the west to the League of the Iroquois in the east, in what is now upstate New York.

The Algonquian languages were closely related, a reflection of the speakers' shared heritage. In the same way, Spanish, Portugese, French, and Italian—the Romance languages of Europe—all are related through a common historical like to the old Roman Empire and its mother tongue, Latin.

Similarly, the Algonquian-speaking people, the most widespread language family in pre-Columbian North America, also grew from a common root. Among Native Americans—whose elders are given respect and for whom a title of age is proof of honor and influence—the Lenni Lenape were known as the "Grandfathers"; they were acknowledged as the progenitor tribe of what the French called the "grand old Algonquian Family."[1] Since so many of the Algonquian-speaking tribes referred to themselves as the "grandchildren" of the Lenni Lenape, the Algonquians might more properly be called the Lenape family.

The Lenni Lenape lived, as did most other woodland tribes, in a confederation of small towns and villages. The Lenni Lenape government was a participatory democracy, with councils presided over by chiefs, known as sachems, whose authority came from their powers of persuasion. As William Penn later commented, "'Tis admirable to consider, how powerful the Kings are, and yet how they move by the Breath of their People."[2]

Ties of kinship among the Lenni Lenape were all-important because they also constituted social and political influence. Like most of the Lenape nations, the Lenni Lenape were bound by family ties. Families made up a village, villages made up a tribe, and tribes combined in larger groups through family connections. Within their vast, extended family, the Lenni Lenape maintained a clear sense of their clan and family lineages. Inheritance among the Lenni Lenape was matriarchal, through the female line, so a man's position was more likely to go to his sister's son than to his own. Besides reflecting the status of women, this custom, so widespread among the Eastern tribes, also had a practical basis: it is easier to identify the mother of a child than the father.

Among the Lenni Lenape, there was a customary division of labor between men and women, but the division was not unequal, and each would lend a hand as needed. Women were not expected to be councilors, but they owned most of the household property and the products of the fields they tended. Men were responsible for clearing the fields and hunting for meat in the forest. Children were loved and valued, and everyone in the village gladly lent a hand in bringing them up to be a part of the community. Elders were universally respected for their wisdom and experience, and every grey hair was considered a badge of honor.

Life revolved around the cycle of the seasons, as reflected in the changes in the Lenni Lenape's woodland home. When spring came, the Lenni Lenape congregated by rapids and waterfalls to gather the spawning fish swarming upstream, hunt bear and deer, and pick strawberries. As summer approached, the people dispersed; some went to the seashore to gather shellfish for food and for shells used in making valuable wampum beads. Most went inland to prepare their garden plots in the soft, deep soil of the river bottoms, clearing fields by charring trees in order to fell them with stone axes, then planting crops of corn, beans, squash, and tobacco in the ash-enriched soil. These fields would last for a generation, after which it would be time to clear new fields or move elsewhere. Summer was the time for tending the plots, gathering fruits, berries, and medicinal herbs, hunting and fishing, and taking trips to trade, explore, and visit relatives. Autumn was the time for group hunts, using fire to drive the game and to clear out the brush under the trees, and for gathering and storing the harvest. In the winter, warm in their fur robes inside their wigwams and bark houses, they would listen to stories and create clothes, weapons, and household items with skill and artistry.

The land where they lived was divided into territories for hunting, fishing, or farming with usage rights understood to be held by particular families, or communally by a particular village. However, this did not constitute owning the land itself, as one could not own the sunlight or the air. It was also considered boorish to deny requests to share usage rights, for hospitality and liberality were paramount to the Lenni Lenape. As William Penn later put it, "Nothing is too good for their friend; give them a fine Gun, Coat, or other thing, it may pass twenty hands, before it sticks; light of Heart, strong Affections, but soon spent: the most merry creatures that live, Feast and Dance almost perpetually; they never have much, nor want much: Wealth circulateth like the Blood, all parts partake; and though none shall want what another hath, yet exact Observers of Property."[3]

The Lenni Lenape were on intimate terms with their environment and with the spirits that give it life through a connection to the infinite. To find that connection for themselves, they paid careful attention to their dreams and visions, and they achieved adulthood by contacting a guardian spirit through a vision quest. People who were exceptionally favored by the spirit world became healers and shamans.

Subordinate manitos or creators were thought to be in charge of all the creatures and natural forces of the world, and everything, from the rocks to the wind, was in some way alive. As a Delaware man told the anthropologist Frank Speck, "All manitos pray, because we hear them sometimes, our grandfathers the trees, joining in earnest prayer when the wind blows through them."[4]

Their religious observances and dances climaxed every year in the Gamwing or Big House Ceremony. This profound ritual, which they believed helped maintain the cosmos, lasted twelve days, and included thanksgiving prayers and the sharing of dreams and visions. It took place in the large ceremonial lodge or "Big House" that was a prominent feature of the typical Lenni Lenape village.

The layout of the Big House was a symbolic representation of the world, with a central column connecting sky and earth, and walls facing the four directions. The Big House of the Eastern Woodland region was similar in design to the Medicine Lodge still found among the Lenape tribes of the Great Lakes area. These ceremonial lodges are analogous to the structure used for the Sun Dance among the Lenape tribes of the Great Plains. The existence of the same type of ritual structure in an area extending from the Atlantic to the Rockies is evidence of the ancient roots shared by the various Lenape cultures.[5]

To Record Their History

Like all of these cultures, the Lenni Lenape kept records of important information with devices that served as aids to memory. With these mnemonic devices, they could recall events and information in surprising detail. Among these devices were wampum strings and belts made of beads that had been laboriously made from certain seashells. Prayer sticks or song sticks, wooden tablets with engraved symbols, were used to record the verses of a sacred song or prayer, or to record other important information such as family history. As the Moravian missionary Loskiel reported, "The Delaware keep geneologies, with the character of each man, if wise, rich, renowned, or a mighty warrior. They use hieroglyphs on wood, trees and stones, to give caution, information, communicate events, achievements, [and] keep records."[6]

One such record is the Wallam Olum or Red Record, the history of the Lenni Lenape and the Lenape family, recorded on a set of song sticks. Its symbols may have come to Rafinesque either on pieces of birch bark or on wood; Rafinesque mentions "wooden originals" on which the symbols were "painted & engraved." He also says "*Olum* . . . implies a record, a notched stick, an engraved piece of wood or bark . . ." If these symbols of the Red Record are as ancient as they appear to be, they probably were originally engraved in wood for permanence. This custom has been described by Chief George Copway of the Ojibwa, grandchildren of the Lenni Lenape. His description serves to explain how such records could endure for generations:

> There is a place where the sacred records are deposited in the Indian country. These records are made on one side of bark and board plates, and are examined once [every] fifteen years, at which time the decaying ones are replaced by new plates . . . The guardians had for a long time selected a most unsuspected spot, where they dug fifteen feet, and sunk large cedar trees around the excavation. In the center was placed a large hollow

cedar log, besmeared at one end with gum. The open end is uppermost, and in it are placed the records, after being enveloped in the down of geese or swans.[7]

Some of the rituals associated with the Red Record have even appeared in a work of fiction. A description of its reading in *Dickon Among the Lenape Indians* by the noted anthropologist Mark Harrington allows us to share in one ritual. In a scene set in precolonial times, during the annual Gamwing or Big House Ceremony, a young white castaway witnesses a recitation of the Red Record in which the chief begins:

> One day, long ago, when our ancestors resided in the North, there lived a man who believed that the story of our people should never be forgotten. Knowing that people are, by nature, forgetful, he tried to plan some way to make them remember. Finally, it is said, a method of doing this was revealed to him in a dream. Truly, he was instructed to prepare flat, wooden tablets and to paint upon them pictures in red which call to mind the things he wished to remember. To begin with, he painted the stories of the first days of the world as they were told by the old men of his time; then, he painted pictures to represent important things as they happened. On his death the tablets and the work were carried on by his family until the present day. You see before you Talking-Wood, the present owner of the set of tablets, which we call Wa' lum O' loom.

After the recitation, the castaway says, "Little-Bear and I squirmed through the crowd and succeeded in getting a glimpse of the tablets before Naked-Bear wrapped them up. They were about two spans long and three fingers wide, and the figures seemed to be scratched into the wood, red paint being rubbed into the scratches."[8]

These "scratches" or engravings are silent testimonials to an amazing story, including an epic migration out of Asia. The Red Record tells the story of the rise of the Lenape family, as seen from the point of view of one core group that later became the Lenni Lenape. In describing the migration of this ancestral group, the Red Record also tells of those who branched off or who were left behind; these people may have founded the other branches of the widespread Lenape tribes.

For those parts of the Red Record that cannot be explained from the surviving recorded traditions of the Lenni Lenape, explanations can usually be found among the recorded traditions of their closest Lenape family relatives—the Mohicans, the Nanticokes, and the Shawnee—or among other related tribes such as the Ojibwa, who, because of their location and their numbers, were able to retain many elements of the aboriginal Lenape culture.

The Red Record parallels many Lenape traditions such as those concerning the origins of the world. Among the myths recorded from the Lenape family members are those dealing with the Mother of Life. Sometimes the Mother of Life is the one who gives birth to the fish, the birds, and the beasts; sometimes this is achieved by the Ancestral Man or directly by the Great Spirit. A legend called "The Corn Mother" from the Penobscots, relatives of the Lenni Lenape from New England, describes the origin of the primordial Man and Woman:

> When Kloskurbeh, the All-maker, lived on earth, there were no people yet. But one day when the sun was high, a youth appeared and called him "Uncle, brother of my mother." This young man was born from the foam of the waves, foam quickened by the wind and warmed by the sun. It was the motion of the wind, the moistness of water, and the sun's warmth which gave him life—warmth above all, because warmth is life. And the young man lived with Kloskurbeh and became his chief helper.
>
> Now, after these two powerful beings had created all manner of things, there came to them, as the sun was shining at high noon, a beautiful girl. She was born of the wonderful earth plant, and of the dew, and of warmth. Because a drop of dew fell on a leaf and was warmed by the sun, and the warming sun is life, this girl came into being—from the green living plant, from moisture, and from warmth.
>
> "I am love," said the young maiden. "I am a strength giver. I am the nourisher, I am the provider of men and animals. They all love me."
>
> Then Kloskurbeh thanked the Great Mystery Above for having sent them the maiden. The youth, the Great Nephew, married her, and the girl conceived and thus became First Mother. And Kloskurbeh, the Great Uncle, who teaches humans all they need to know, taught their children how to live. Then he went away to dwell in the north, from which he will return sometime when he is needed.[9]

The corruption of a golden age is also featured in aboriginal Lenni Lenape tradition, along with the symbolism of a snake as a force of potential misfortune. (All of these Lenape myths arose independently of the Biblical story of the Garden of Eden [see page 175].) The Lenni Lenape had a strong belief in the powers of magic, and the tales of blessings gone awry may reflect the age-old dilemma of how to use great

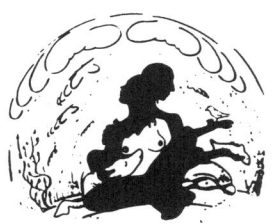

Primordial couple. Pictured here is a conception of the primordial creative couple, bringing forth the plants and animals.

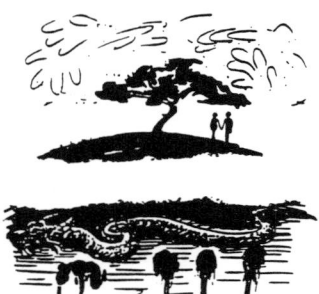

Corruption scene.
Pictured here is an
impression of the end of
the first age, as described
in the Red Record.

power only for good, for white magic and black magic are but two sides of the same coin, just as iron can be used to make either a plowshare or a sword.

The Lenape myth of the Flood may seem to owe something to the Bible because the two versions are so similar, however, the ethnologist Emerson points out, "it should be recalled that in the 1600's the Indians expressed astonishment at the likeness to the Jesuit Fathers, who resented the comparison as an indignity and a sacrilege."[10] Apparently, the Indians thought the influence was the other way around. The Lenape myth of the great Water Monster and the Flood was recorded as early as 1634 by the Jesuit Father LeJeune. This myth is told in many versions among the Lenape tribes. The basic story as told by the Lenni Lenape and recorded by Reverend John Heckewelder agrees in most particulars with the version in the Red Record.[11]

The account of the Flood in the Red Record concludes with the re-creation of the world on the back of a great turtle. This tradition was recorded as early as 1679, when the Dutch travelers Donkers and Sluyter reported the belief of the New Jersey Delawares that the world was brought forth upon a giant tortoise, who created according to the wishes of a primal deity. The primal deity may represent the Creative Hero known as Nenabush, who represents the active principle, the energy of life, which is also represented by light.[12] The turtle, on the other hand, is usually used by Native Americans as a symbolic bearer of Mother Earth, who brings forth the forms containing this energy.[13] The Lenni Lenape referred to North America, as did most Native Americans, as Turtle Island.

In almost every Lenape account of the Flood, the restoration of the world on the back of the Turtle is accomplished using mud brought up by a diving creature. In the version told by the Ojibwa, the beaver is the first to try to reach the bottom of the water to fetch the needed bit of earth. It dies in the attempt, but is revived by Nenabash. Then the otter tries and fails. Then, as all hope is fading, the lowly muskrat tries, and finally comes up dead, but with the precious bit of earth in its paws. Nenabush then grows the new world from this seed, through a magic song and a magic dance.[14]

Nenabush was well known under many names and incarnations as the Culture Hero of the Lenape people. To the Abenaki Confederacy he was known as Glooskap; to the Massachusetts he was the Common Father; to the Cree he was Wisakketcjak, the Trickster; while to the Blackfoot he was Napi, the Old Man. He also was known as a prankster and as a Cosmic Fool. His association in the Red Record with the Hare was also common in native tradition, and may be connected to a symbolic meaning as the Bringer of Life.[15]

In myths such as the stories of Nenabush and the Flood, creating and changing the world is shown to be possible by the power of prayer, as proof that the spirits will respond to those in real need. So the story of the Flood is also a metaphor for the vision quest in which a Lenape youth would hope to find a guiding spirit through fasting, hardship, and prayer.

Nenabush, the Great Hare, the shaper of the world, is still not finished with his creation, but constantly walks around and around, increasing it and changing things here and there. Nenabush, as a great hero, has the ability to create and metamorphosize at will. He can give help in dreams, and is a great inventor, teacher, and benefactor. The nature of this great Hero is full of contradictions. He is often called the Great Hare or the Great Light by the Native Americans, but he also has his all-too-human characteristics. Like Bugs Bunny or Brer Rabbit, he can also be a great practical joker, and sometimes gets entangled in his own schemes. Nenabush is often bawdy and outrageous, and the stories of his pranks and adventures are always popular among Native American audiences.

The Asian Roots of the Red Record

In addition to Lenape origin myths, the Red Record also includes historical data from distant times and places. It is, in fact, remarkable how the story told in the Red Record parallels what we now know about the development of society in Asia in the distant past.

A great change took place in the Paleolithic Age with the development of new kinds of stone points capable of killing even the largest animals. As the anthropoligist Louis A. Brennan describes what happened, "So confident were the Paleo-hunters of the efficacy of their new stone-tipped weapons that they did a daring thing: they left the fixed locale they had been scrounging over, where they knew every turtle pond and rabbit hole, and committed themselves to the shifting environment of the big-game herds."[16] Hard-working and ingenious, these hunters prospered, living off the herds in the plains of Eastern Siberia, following the interconnecting waterways northward through the endless taiga forests. The consistency of the environment encouraged the hunters to spread far and wide.

The Red Record describes how this expansion brought the ancestors of the Lenape into conflict with their enemies, the Snakes. The Red Record tells how the Snakes in the northeast fled before the Lenape hunters. The conflict between the Lenape and the Snakes recalls the ancient conflict between the proto-Chinese and the "barbarians" to the North, among them tribes they called the Turtle People. A possibility of contact between the proto-Chinese and the proto-Lenape is suggested by resemblances, both in form and in content, between many ideographic symbols in the Red Record and the oldest form of writing known to

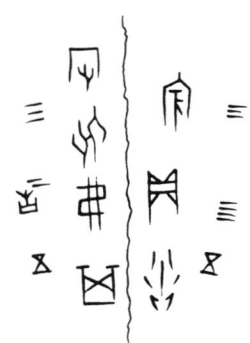

Bone oracle symbols.
Examples of bone oracle
script, carved on either
side of a seam in a turtle
shell, are shown here.

China, Pre-Shang Dynasty Bone Oracle Script, which was first described in 1899. This ancient form of writing was carved into ox scapulas or the shells of giant tortoises. Heat was then applied to cause cracks in the bone or shell, and thus reveal the answer to the carved question. Several researchers, including those in the Indiana Historical Society study, have noted the resemblance.[17] The distinguished Chinese scholar Dr. Chen Chi-yun also compared the ancient form of writing to the symbols in the Red Record. He noted the similar expressions for even abstract concepts such as the soul and said, "The parallels are striking to say the least."[18]

Traditional Lenape legends also seem to describe the explorations that led to the momentous crossing from Asia into America described in the Red Record. A Shawnee legend describing an exploration of the New World was recorded from the story of an aged Shawnee at Piqua in Ohio in 1823. It describes in great detail an ancient Arctic home, and how and why their ancestors crossed the ocean, which in the legend is called the Great Salt Lake. This legend was given the unusual title of "Pomatare, the Flying Beaver" by J.A. Jones in his *Traditions of the North American Indians*.[19] "Pomatare" can be loosely translated as "The Explorers," and the rest of the title may well refer to Head Beaver and Great Bird, who are described in the Red Record as being the leaders of the journey to the New World. The legend tells of explorers led by a Man-Fish on a long canoe journey that lasts for two and a half moons. The explorers travel to a rich shore with mountains whose summits shoot flames into the sky. The inhabitants of this "happy hunting ground" run from the visitors. The explorers have an encounter with a Man-Goat, a being who may have been wearing an elaborate mask in the manner of the people of the Northwest Coast, who eventually leads them to find a new home.

The traditions of the Lenni Lenape, as recorded by Heckewelder in a later time when they were known as the Delaware Indians, state that their ancestors came out of a land of ice and snow in the far northwest of the continent.[20] Other traditions of their closest relatives—the Nanticokes, the Shawnee, and the Mohicans—give even more detail, including what may be descriptions of the actual crossing of the Bering Strait itself.

The words and symbols in the Red Record make it clear that this crossing was accomplished on a bridge of ice. This is echoed by a Nanticoke legend, as recorded in 1767 by the missionary Charles Beatty who wrote, "They came to a great water. One of the Indians that went before them tried the depth of it by a long pole or reed, which he had in his hand, and found it too deep for them to wade. Upon their being non-plussed, and not knowing how to get over it, their God made a bridge over the water in one night, and the next morning, after they were all over, God took away the bridge."[21]

The Shawnees also remembered this momentous event. They told how, in the words of Brinton, ". . . at some indefinitely remote past, they had arrived at the main land after crossing a wide water. Their ancestors succeeded in this by their great control of magic arts, their occult power enabling them to walk over the water as if it had been land. Until within the present century [the 1800's] this legend was repeated annually, and a yearly sacrifice offered up in memory of their safe arrival."[22]

The Mohicans, as closely related to the Lenni Lenape on the north as the Nanticokes and Shawnee were on the south, also recalled this event, according to Brinton. The Mohicans' description reflects the strong currents characteristic of the Bering Strait, as well as its abundant marine life, with great numbers of whales migrating between the Arctic Ocean and the Pacific Ocean. Brinton writes, ". . . their early forefathers came out of the northwest, forsaking a tide-water country and crossing over a great watery tract, called *ukhok-pek* ('snake water,' or 'water where snakes are abundant') . . . They crossed many streams, but none in which the water ebbed and flowed, until they reached the Hudson."[23]

Even the Cheyennes, a Lenape tribe of the Great Plains, may have a version of this story. In an extraordinary legend, they recall:

> . . . having lived in a land that was perpetually covered with ice and snow. Trying to escape the continual rule of *Hoimaha* [the winter storm], they started eastward toward the sun. After many years, they came to a narrow neck of sea at a time when the water was frozen. As the people were about halfway across the frozen water, one of the young women discovered a horn sticking out of the ice.
>
> The horn took her fancy. Even in these difficult times of moving, the women and the children made sliding sticks from horns and managed to enjoy life a little more. The woman wanted this horn, for it was large and long, and would make a splendid sliding stick. She tried to pull the horn out of the ice, but the harder she pulled, the tighter the horn seemed to be imbedded. Finally, she called to her relatives for assistance. Some of the men came and helped her. But, like her, they were unable to pull the horn out. Then, they began to cut the horn, for they liked the girl and wanted to make her happy. As they cut deeper into the horn, blood spurted out in great gushes.
>
> The people were frightened and grouped together on both sides of the men who had been cutting the horn. Just as they realized that the horn must be that of a monster, they felt a great tremor and knew that the monster must be struggling below the frozen water. Before anyone could move away, the ice suddenly broke, the horn disappeared, and a great chasm

appeared. Some of the people were drowned. Many of them found themselves before an ever-widening channel of water, so they had to retreat to the land from whence they had come. Those on the side toward the Sun watched their friends retreat; then, saddened by the insuperable gulf between them, they took flight onward in pursuit of the Sun and moved into the East and the New Land. Never have these people—the *Tsi-Tsi-Tsas* [Cheyenne]—forgotten this story.[24]

O.M. Spencer, who lived among the Shawnees around 1792, reported the common belief in another "happy hunting ground" that lay to the west, beyond the ocean.[25] Although this might refer to the Native American version of heaven, it might also include some ancestral memory of a first hunting ground that did indeed lie beyond the western ocean, in Asia.

A Process of Corruption and Rebirth

Once in the New World, the ancestors of the Lenape are described in the Red Record as gradually migrating southeastward, along both sides of the Canadian Rockies. This led one group along what is now known as the Northwest Coast, where Ayamek, the Seizer (IV:15–16) conquered all the enemy tribes. After Ayamek, there was a time of great evil events lasting for the reign of ten unnamed chiefs (IV:17). Following this perod of evil came a succession of other chiefs who gradually healed and reunited the tribe by setting examples of virtue.

This process of corruption and rebirth is reflected in stories about the origins of two of the most ancient and profound religious features of the Lenni Lenape, the Big House Ceremony and the Mising Mask, which may reach back to this time.

In the version told by the Delaware spiritual leader Charles Elkhair and reported by Harrington, three mistreated boys were once aided in their extremity by a vision of Mising, the Keeper of the Game, riding on an elk. He took one of the boys on an adventure to the nearby mystic mountains, which are described as running from the north to the south. Meanwhile, the evil ways of the Lenape continued, and they neglected the crucial ceremonies of thanksgiving and vision-sharing for ten years. Finally the wrath of the Great Spirit erupted in violent earthquakes, featuring hot oil gushing from the ground, which lasted for twelve moons. The terrified people crowded into the great house of the chief to pray for help. Mising appeared to the boys and told them to dress like him with a suit of fur, a rattle and a mask of red and black halves, and to bring everyone at harvest time to the great house. There the penitent people all were given the instructions for the Gamwing, the Big House Ceremony of sharing and worship, which they were warned never to neglect, for it helped to maintain the cosmos. Through the ceremony, they regained the favor of the Great Spirit, and Mising has been their helper ever since.[26] The Lenni Lenape or Delawares continued to annually conduct the Big House Ceremony well into the twentieth century. The last time was to pray for the safety of Delaware men fighting in World War II. All returned unhurt.

With the Big House Ceremony a part of their lives, the Lenape continued south into the Great Plateau. Here, the Red Record says, they first learned how to grow crops until drought drove them to the eastward, onto the Great Plains. The later stage of the Lenape journey across the North American continent is described in detail in Delaware legends recorded by Hecke-welder.

"The Expedition of the Lenni Lenape" was recorded by Heckewelder in 1799. This legend tells how long ago, in the shadow of the Rocky Mountains, a vision of a journey into the East, to a beautiful land beyond the Appalachians, came in a dream to a young chief named Wangewaha, The Hard Heart. Upon being told of this vision, the head priest and the elders undertook a fast to learn the will of the Almighty. After three days, the Great Spirit spoke to them, and gently urged them to make the journey. Accordingly, the greater part of the nation made ready to go, packing the bones of their ancestors onto the dog sleds, along with dried corn and pemmican (a meat patty prepared by pounding dried meat into a paste and mixing it with fat and berries).

To protect the Lenape from any enemies, the shamans made a powerful war medicine by mixing the ashes of the bones of a terrifying wildcat of ancient times with pieces of the horns of the great Snake of the Waters, an old rattlesnake who had received a Lenape maiden as his bride in return for his services. Following the rattlesnake's directions, they then made their way to the Medicine Stone, where they made peace with all of the Snake tribe, and continued on into the unknown East. (The Lenape often referred to human enemies as Snakes; the Red Record tells of many battles with the Snakes prior to the eastward migration.)

Out on the Plains, far from their old home, the travelers encountered a powerful tribe of strangers. Fearlessly, the Lenape ambassador, Mottschujinga or Little Grizzly Bear, went to meet them, nude in the ancient manner, carrying in one hand a black wampum belt containing a declaration of war, and in the other hand a Pipe of Peace. He waited for the strangers to make their choice. The choice was for peace, and these strangers, the Iroquois, became friends and allies of the Lenape, and promised to help them if the need arose. The Lenape then traveled on into the East, where their destiny awaited them.[27]

In the Red Record, it is told that the Lenape found the people called the Talegas occupying the land east of the Mississippi. In his book *History, Manners and Customs of the Indian Nations*, Heckewelder includes a rare description of these mysterious people, better known as the Moundbuilders, in a report of the ancient migration of the Lenni Lenape, as told to him by the Delawares, "according to the traditions handed down to them by their ancestors."

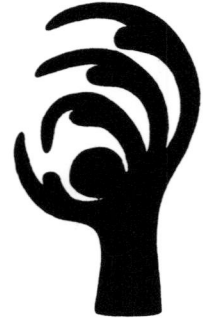

Talega design.
The author has redrawn a Moundbuilder design of a bird's claw, which was originally cut from a sheet of mica.

> The spies which the Lenape had sent forward for the purpose of reconnoitering, had long before their arrival discovered that the country to the east of the Mississippi was inhabited by a very powerful nation, who had many large towns built on the great rivers flowing through the land. These people (as I was told) called themselves Tallegwi or Talligewi . . . Many wonderful things are told of this famous people. They are said to have been remarkably tall and stout, and there are traditions that there were giants among them. It is related, that they had built to themselves regular fortifications or entrenchments, from whence they would sally out . . .

Heckewelder goes on to describe the outbreak of the Talega War, in an account that parallels the Red Record:

> When the Lenape arrived on the banks of the Mississippi, they sent a message to the Alligewi [Talegas], to request permission to settle themselves in their neighborhood. This was denied them, but they obtained leave to pass through the country, and seek a settlement further to the eastward. They accordingly commenced passing the Mississippi, when the Alligewi discovering their great numbers became alarmed, and made a furious attack on those who had crossed. Fired at their treachery, the Lenape consulted on what was to be done; whether to retreat, or to try their strength on their oppressors. While this was going on the Mengwe [Iroquois], who had contented themselves with looking on at a distance, offered to join the Lenape, upon condition that they should be entitled to a share of the country in case the combination was successful.[28]

The proposal was accepted, and the allies attacked the Talegas. The struggle was long and hard. The Red Record says that four chiefs came and went before the last of the Talega strongholds was captured, whereupon the Talegas fled down the Mississippi River, never to return.

After the Talega War, the victors divided up the Talega country. Both the Red Record and Heckewelder describe the Iroquois taking the territory around the Great Lakes, and the Lenape settling to the south, along the Ohio River. The Red Record mentions a brief falling out between the allies, but as Book V begins, "All was peaceful, long ago, there in the Talega Country (V:1)." After many generations of peace and growth have passed, the Red Record tells of the journey of Onowutok, the Prophet, "West, to those left behind (V:13)." Heckewelder in his traditional history confirms that "a portion of their people remained beyond the Mississippi," and describes in an account that continues to parallel the Red Record how a major portion of the Lenape went eastward on the final stage of their migration:

> Ultimately some of the more adventurous among them crossed the mountains towards the rising sun, and falling on streams running to the eastward, followed them to the great Bay River (Susquehanna) and thence to the Bay (Chesapeake) itself. As they pursued their travels, partly by land and partly by water . . . they discovered the great river which we call the Delaware; and still further to the eastward, the *Scheyichbi* country, now called New Jersey. Afterwards they reached the stream now called the Hudson. The reports of the adventurers caused large bodies to follow them, who settled upon the four great rivers, the Delaware, Hudson, Susquehanna and Potomac, making the Delaware, which they call *Linapewihittuck* (the river of the Lenape) the center of their possessions.[29]

The Red Record describes how the Lenape prospered in their new home. Another chief named Tamanend arose to bring all of the Lenape together in friendship. Soon after this period, the first European explorers appeared. (Heckewelder's retelling of this first, tragicomic encounter is presented on pages 140-144.)

Following this, the Red Record tells of several sachems whose names seem to refer to incidents in Delaware legends recorded by Richard Adams.[30] White Otter (V:44) may refer to Mekehappa, an ugly outcast who, with the aid of beneficent spirits, was able to bag a sacred white otter, thereby winning the hand of a powerful chief's daughter so that eventually he would become chief. The holy man White Horn (V:45) may refer to a sacred tusk kept among the Lenni Lenape, taken from a sleeping giant bear that was supposed to have great magic powers. And Cranberry Eating (V:49) refers to the old legend of the color of cranberries, which was supposed to be from the blood of the animals who died trying to stop the last mastodon, who was raging in rebellion against the will of the Great Spirit.

The Red Record also notes how the growth of the Lenape people led to their division into many parts. According to Heckewelder's traditional history:

> The largest portion [of the Lenape people] they supposed, settled on the Atlantic. [These] were divided into three tribes, two of which were distinguished as *Unamis*, or Turtle, and *Unalachtigo* or Turkey. These chose the lands lying nearest the coast. Their settlements extended from the *Mahicanittuck* (river of the Mohicans, or Hudson) to beyond the Potomac . . . The third great tribe, the *Minsi* [Munsees] . . . or tribe of the wolf, lived back of the others, forming a kind of bulwark, and watching the nations of the *Mengwe* [Iroquois of the Six Nations]. They were considered the most active and warlike of all the tribes. . . .[31]

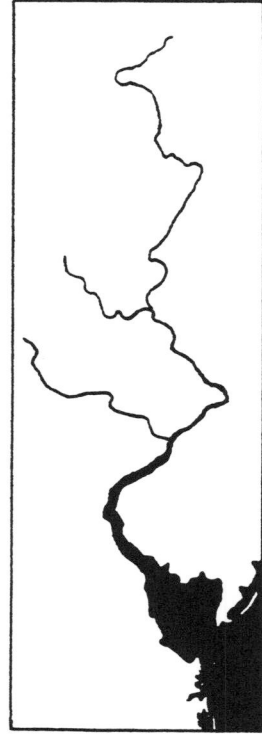

Delaware River.
The Lenni Lenape spread out along the length of the Delaware River.

The Wolf, Turtle, and Turkey tribes (also called clans) have continued among the Delawares to the present day. Each name refers back to an ancestral totem. The Turtles or "Shufflers" are regarded as the oldest group, and represent all hairless creatures; the Wolves were nicknamed the "Paws," and represent hairy creatures; and the Turkeys or "Scratchers" are regarded as the youngest, and represent creatures with feathers.[32]

The other names for the divisions, however, are more likely geographical, rather than geneological, in nature. According to Brinton, the Munsees were the "mountaineers" living at the headwaters of the Delaware, and "Unami" meant the "people down the river." The third division, which Heckewelder called the Unalachtigo, was the "people near the ocean."[33]

In concluding his account of the Lenape's traditional history, Heckewelder says, "From the above three divisions or tribes, comprising the body of the people called Delawares, sprung many others, who, having for their own convenience chosen distant spots to settle in, and increasing in numbers, gave themselves names, or received them from others. Thus they formed separate and distinct tribes, yet did not deny their origin, but retained their affection for the parent tribe, of which they were even proud to be called the grandchildren."[34]

Generation after generation passed. The Red Record concludes with the Lenni Lenape masters of their world, at the head of a great extended family of tribes, in the forest home of their dreams. Their culture was strong, and they were proud to carry on the traditions of their ancestors. Beneath the majestic trees, the young would eagerly gather to hear the wisdom of their elders, and learn again how to recite the sacred story of the past.

Part Two

The Red Record

Chapter 4

Presenting
the Red Record

The Wallam Olum, the Red Record, is unique as a record of American antiquity. Its symbols and words open the door to a previously lost age of our past, and enable us to see the Lenni Lenape's discovery of America through their own eyes.

The original Delaware words presented here are taken directly from the Rafinesque Manuscript. Those words that are only partially legible in the Manuscript are given the spelling found in the Indiana Historical Society study. When an unambiguous translation could not be determined, the original Lenape word appears in the translation.

The symbols shown here are improved renderings based directly on those in the Rafinesque Manuscript, which were originally drawn by Rafinesque with indifferent care. Apparently, they were sketches of the original symbols that have since been lost. Shapes that are obviously meant to be geometrically regular are shown lopsided and uneven: circles are irregular, straight lines are crooked and tilted, and lines vary greatly in thickness because of the quill pens Rafinesque was using. Yet these sketches still hint at the graphic power of the symbols. Like logos, they grow in effectiveness when they are drawn with care and conviction. The geometric elements of the symbols are drawn more accurately in this version, which at the same time preserves the overall size, proportions, and non-geometric details found in Rafinesque's originals.

The symbols are arranged here in a reconstruction of their probable arrangement on the missing record tablets. Clues provided by Rafinesque as well as examples of other Lenape carved records give an idea of how the lost Red Record tablets may have appeared.

The Rafinesque Manuscript divides the Red Record into five sections, which are usually referred to as "books." In Rafinesque's publication of the account in *The American Nations*, he called each of the first three books a separate "song," and further subdivided the fourth book into four songs of sixteen verses each, and the fifth and final book into three songs of twenty verses each. These sixteen-verse and twenty-verse divisions are indicated in the Rafinesque Manuscript. Could these represent the division of the symbols onto the original tablets?

Most of the Red Record is very regular in form: four words per verse in Book IV, three words per verse in Book V, so it seems reasonable to suppose that the tablets were divided regularly as well. Having all the tablets the same size and shape would make them easier to bundle and keep together as a set.

The standard dimensions of a tablet can be determined by a layout of the symbols that may have appeared upon it. The size of these symbols is determined by Rafinesque's drawings, the best available guide. The symbols are given a consistent vertical orientation, which is unusual among Lenape pictographs in general, but not uncommon among prayer sticks. Sometimes these prayer sticks, such as the Kickapoo example being read by Cock Turkey in the frontispiece, have an ornamental shape with outsize additions at each end. Rafinesque, however, makes no mention of such a shape, and there is no pattern of outsized symbols such as would be found in these enlarged ends; a better fit of the symbols into the tablets comes from a simple rectangular shape.

If sixteen symbols appeared on each tablet of Book IV and twenty for each tablet of Book V, then this would create a tablet length that would be unusually long for a Lenape song stick. In addition, this standard length would not yield even divisions for the symbols of Book I and Book III. For each of these two books, at least two tablets would be required, and the symbols upon each tablet would have to be scattered, with a spacing far wider than elsewhere. The solution is a tablet of half this length.

Tracings from Rafinesque's drawings of the symbols show that they could all fit very comfortably on twenty-two tablets measuring roughly 7 inches (17.78 cm) long by 2 inches (5.08 cm) wide, having ten symbols per tablet in Book V, eight per tablet in Book IV, and irregular numbers

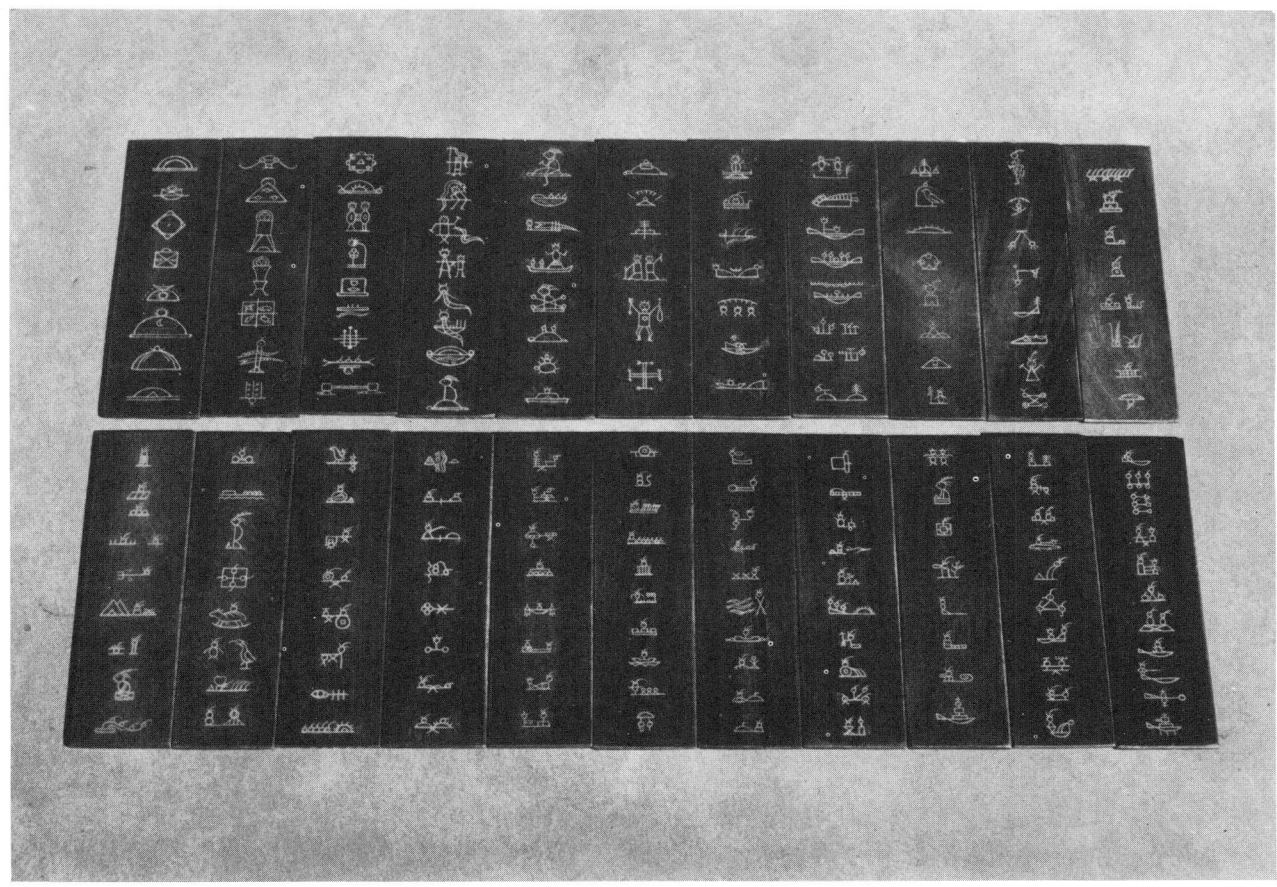

Figure 4.1. A replica set of Wallam Olum tablets carved by the author. There are three tablets for Book I, two for Book II, three for Book III, eight for Book IV, and six for Book V. Each tablet is 7 inches long and 2 inches wide.

in Books I, II, and III. There are, therefore, three tablets to Book I, two for Book II, three for Book III, eight for Book IV, and six for Book V. These parameters were used to carve the replica set of tablets seen in Figure 4.1.

On pages 51 to 139, the Wallam Olum, the Red Record, is presented in its traditional five books, further subdivided according to these probable tablet divisions. Each portion of the account represented by a tablet is called a "chapter," and each of these chapters has been given a descriptive title suggested by its content.

In keeping with accounts that describe the symbols as being painted and in accordance with the usual translation of "Wallam" as "Red," the symbols are reproduced in red, a favorite color among the Lenni Lenape, who regarded it as sacred. The symbols are shown on the left-hand page between the original Delaware words and a new English translation. The criteria for this new translation are: the closest possible matching of the original sense of both the words and symbols, considered together; agreement of the translated account with native traditions; readability and logical flow; and matching wherever possible the number of syllables in the English words with the number of syllables in the original Delaware words.

On the right-hand pages are a descriptive title for the chapter, and its retelling in a form closer to a narrative, with interpretations based on tribal traditions and analysis of the chapter's words and symbols. Books III, IV, and V also include original illustrations of the action, and maps giving approximate locations for the incidents of the story, based upon the reconstruction of the migration route as detailed in the Appendix. On the maps, the stages of the migration are shown, with successive population centers shown as circles, and movements as arrows.

I hope this presentation of the Red Record will help bring back some of the vividness and meaning that it held for its original audience. But it must be kept in mind that these words were once the lyrics of a song, a song that is now sung in silence, to a melody we can only imagine.

The Wallam Olum

Book I

Symbols	Original Words	Translation
	1 Sayewitalli Wemiguma Wokgetaki	At the beginning, The sea everywhere Covered the earth.
	2 Hackung-kwelik Owanaku Wak yutali Kitanitowit-essop	Above extended A swirling cloud, And within it, The Great Spirit moved.
	3 Sayewis Hallemewis Nolemewi Elemamik Kitanitowit-essop	Primordial, Everlasting, Invisible, Omnipresent— The Great Spirit moved.
	4 Sohalawak Kwelik Hakik Owak Awasagamak	Bringing forth The sky, The earth, The clouds, The heavens.
	5 Sohalawak Gishuk Nipahum Alankwak	Bringing forth The day, The night, The stars.
	6 Wemi-sohalawak Yulik Yuch-aan	Bringing forth all Of these to move in harmony.
	7 Wich-owagan Kshakan Moshakwat Kwelik Kshipehelep	Stirred to action Strong winds blew, Clearing The sky In rapid streams.
	8 Opeleken Mani-menak Delsin-epit	Pure as snow Arose the lands To be inhabited.

Genesis

Book I: verses 1 through 8

The Wallam Olum, the Red Record, opens with an account of the great myth of Creation, an account that is generally consistent with other recorded Lenape and Native American versions. It begins with primoridal waters covering the world, a characteristic of creation myths everywhere in aboriginal North America except among the Eskimos.[1] From out of the deep came a mist, and within it moved the Creator, the Great Spirit, eternal and omnipresent (I:1–4). The will of the Great Spirit brought forth the sky, the heavens, and the heavenly bodies, all moving in harmony (I:5–6). The mists and waters that covered the earth were blown away, and the land emerged, shining clean (I:7–8).

The Great Spirit was usually referred to by the Lenni Lenape as being male; however, the Shawnee, their close Lenape family relatives, referred to the Great Spirit as "Grandmother."[2] The symbol for I:3 has the same meaning here as in other examples of Lenape-Algonquian pictographs. It was generally used as the symbol for God and the Earth; to the Ojibwa it also meant "Great Spirit; everywhere."[3]

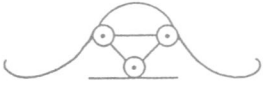

9   Lappinup   Again,
      Kitanitowit   The Great Spirit
      Manito   Created:
      Manitoak   The creator spirits,

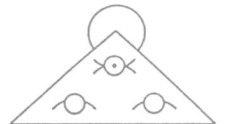

10   Owiniwak   Living beings,
      Angelatawiwak   Immortals,
      Chichankwak   The Souls [for]
      Wemiwak   Everything.

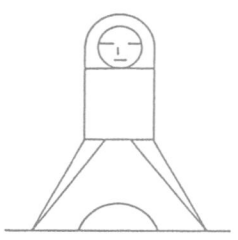

11   Wtenkmanito   Then the Spirit
      Jinwis   Ancestor,
      Lennowak   Grandfather
      Mukom   Of Men,

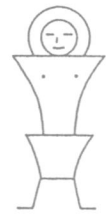

12   Milap   Gave
      Netami-gaho   The First Mother,
      Owini-gaho   Mother of Life,

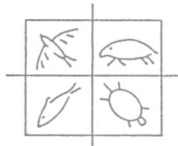

13   Namesik milap   [Who] gave the fish,
      Tulpewik milap   Gave the turtles,
      Awesik milap   Gave the beasts,
      Cholensak milap   Gave the birds.

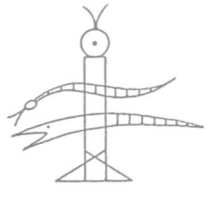

14   Makimani-shak   But the bad spirit
      Sohalawak   Brought forth
      Makowini   Bad creatures:
      N'akowak   The snakes and
      Amangamek   Sea monsters.

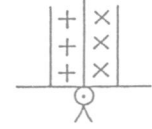

15   Sohalawak   It brought forth
      Uchewak   Flies;
      Sohalawak   It brought forth
      Pungusak   Mosquitos.

The Creation of Life

Book I: verses 9 through 15

The Creator then created the spirits of life—the manitos—and immortal souls for all living things (I:9–10). The belief in immortal spirits inhabiting the mortal bodies of animal and even plant life is also characteristic of Native American tradition. Manito, the word for Spirit, is similar to the Lenape verb *maniton*, which means "to make."[4]

Then the Creator created the Ancestral Man and the Mother of Life, who gave the earth the creatures of the air, land, and water (I:11–13). During the Gamwing, the Big House Ceremony, this story of Creation was often recited, using wampum beads to count off the many gifts of the Creator.[5]

It is unclear here whether these living things were brought forth by the Mother of Life, the Ancestral Man, or even the Great Spirit directly; Lenape myths exist for all three versions. But the Mother of Life seems to be the most likely choice. Note the resemblance in the juxtaposition of Her symbol (I:12) with the cross-like arrangement of animals to which she has given birth (I:13) and the symbol of the Hunter (III:5) with the cross-like directions of His hunts (III:6).

One of the manitos is a spirit of ill will, who creates serpents and sea monsters, flies, and mosquitos (I:14–15). The forces hostile to humans were often symbolized in Lenape myths and stories by horned water snakes and water in general.[6] This spirit's creation of annoying insects recalls the name of one of the chief demons of the Hebrew tradition, Beelzebub, which means "Lord of the Flies."

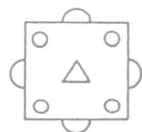

16 Nitisak   Friends were
  Wemi owini   All living things
  W'delsinewuap With each other.

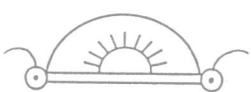

17 Kiwis Wunand The Benefactor
  Wishimanitowak And the helpful spirits
  Essopak   Were busy.

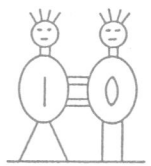

18 Nijini   Those ancestors,
  Netami lennowak The first men,
  Nigoha   Were alone;
  Netami okwewi The first women
  Nantinéwak   Were brought them.

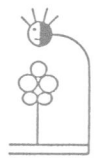

19 Gattamin   Hungry for
  Netami mitzi The first food,
  Nijini   Those ancestors
  Nantiné   Gathered it.

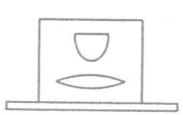

20 Wemi wingi-namenep All were delighted,
  Wemi ksin-elendamep All were carefree,
  Wemi wullatemanuwi All were happy.

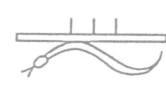

21 Shukand   But then,
  Eli-kemi   Very secretly
  Mekenikink   At the end,
  Wakon   An evil snake,
  Powako   A sorcerer,
  Init'ako   Came to the earth.

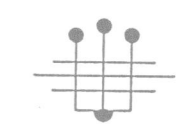

22 Mattalogas   Wickedness,
  Pallalogas   Wrongfulness,
  Maktaten owagan Criminal acts—
  Payat-chik yutali These came there.

23 Maktapan payat Black weather came,
  Wihillan payat Sickness came,
  Mboagan payat Death came.

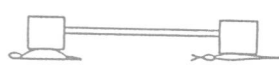

24 Wonwemi   All of this
  Wiwunch   Was long ago
  Kamik atak   In the land beyond
  Kitahikan   The great flood,
  Netamaki   The first world
  Epit   There was.

The Coming of Corruption

Book I: verses 16 through 24

At first, everything was peaceful and happy, with all living things in harmony with one another (I:16), helped and guided by the beneficence of the Great Spirit (I:17). The spirits took care of the people's needs, bringing women to the first men, and providing food for them to gather (I:17–19). Everyone was pleased and contented (I:20). But eventually a serpent, a secret presence of misfortune, grew powerful, causing crime and disharmony (I:21–22). Storms, sickness, and death came into the world (I:23). In the final symbol (I:24), note the split between the Turtle and Snake nations, which foreshadows the Flood and the subsequent wars against the Snakes characteristic of the history of the Lenape.

Tales of the corruption of a golden age abound in world literature. The Delaware belief in a golden age is documented by Heckewelder in a manuscript that tells of long ago, when everyone lived in peace, prosperity, and happiness, and death came only from extreme old age. But this happy time was brought to a close "by the advent of certain evil beings who taught men to kill each other by sorcery."[7]

Book II

Symbols		Original Words	Translation
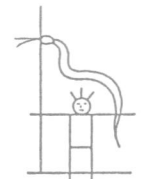	1	Wulamo Maskanako-anup Lennowak Makowini essopak	Long ago, In the time of the Mighty 　Serpent, Were the men, [and] Evil beings.
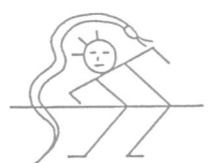	2	Maskanako Shigalusit Nijini essopak Shawelendamep Eken shingalan	The Mighty Serpent Was an enemy to Those ancestors there, Who soon grew To hate it.
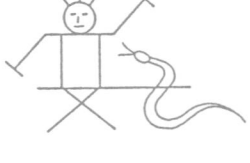	3	Nishawi palliton Nishawi machiton Nishawi matta 　lungundowin	They both fought, They both did wrong, They both had no peace.
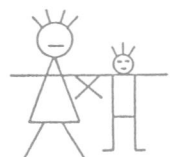	4	Mattapewi wiki Nihantuwit Mekwazoan	Homes were destroyed By murderers And bloodshed.
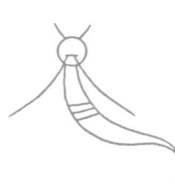	5	Maskanako Gishi penauwelendamep Lennowak Owini Palliton	The Mighty Serpent, Resolving that Men and Living things Be destroyed,
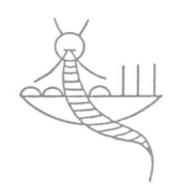	6	Nakowa petonep Amangam petonep Akopehella petonep	Brought the snakes, Brought the sea monsters, Brought the snaking Flood
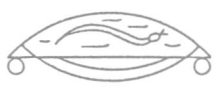	7	Pahella pahella Pohoka pohoka Eshohok eshohok Palliton palliton	Flooding and flooding, Filling and filling, Smashing and smashing, Drowning and drowning.
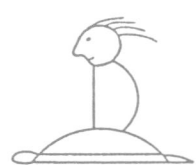	8	Tulapit menapit Nanaboush Maskaboush Owinimokom Linowimokom	At Turtle Island Was Nenabush The great hare, Grandfather to Life, Grandfather of humanity.

The Deluge

Book II: verses 1 through 8

This section of the Red Record tells of the battle against the water monster and of the Flood, a story told in many versions among the Algonquian-speaking tribes. The Lenni Lenape version, as recorded by Heckewelder, agrees in most particulars with what is presented here.[8]

It was the time of the Mighty Serpent (II:1). Men recognized it as a mortal enemy (II:2) and fought unceasingly against it (II:3). Crime and murder increased (II:4). At last, the Serpent resolved to wipe out the men and all living things (II:5) and unleashed the great Flood (II:6), smashing and drowning all things everywhere (II:7).

The Serpent is represented in II:5–6 with horns and whiskers, an interesting parallel with the Chinese image of the Dragon, a snakelike creature also symbolically connected with the water. Other evil beings, allied with the Serpent, seem to be involved here; they are implied in the words of II:1 and shown in the symbol for II:4. In this symbol, the enemy beings have the four-line headdress of the first ancestors of I:18–19, but no eyes, like the face of the Serpent in the two following verses. The men, on the other hand, are shown with the three-line headdress representing the ancestors of the Lenape found in Book III. So this symbol suggests a primordial battle between the corrupted successors of the original humans of Book I, and the uncorrupted element that later became the Lenape of Book III.

There is, however, a note of optimism: an island amidst the

Flood unleashed by the Serpent. On this floating Turtle was Nenabush, the Great Hare, the Grandfather of Men (II:8). In Lenape tradition, the Turtle symbolizes adaptability to either land or water; Nenabush is well known under many names and incarnations as the creative hero of the Lenape people. His identification with the Hare symbolizes a role as the Bringer of Life.[9]

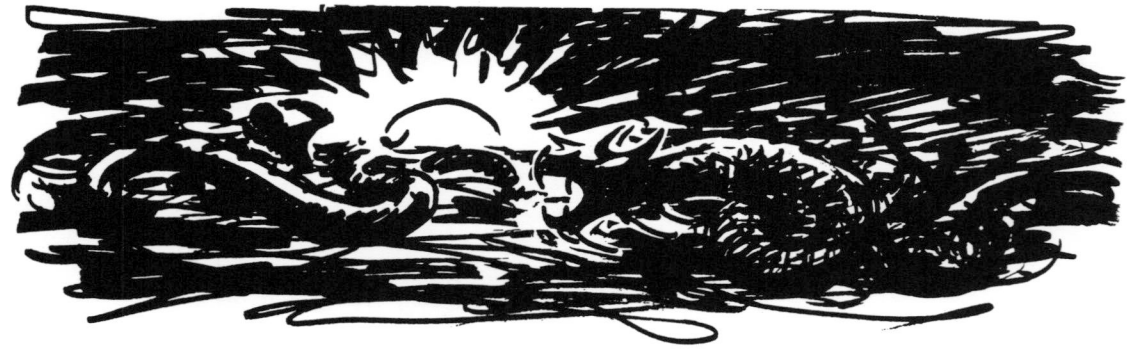

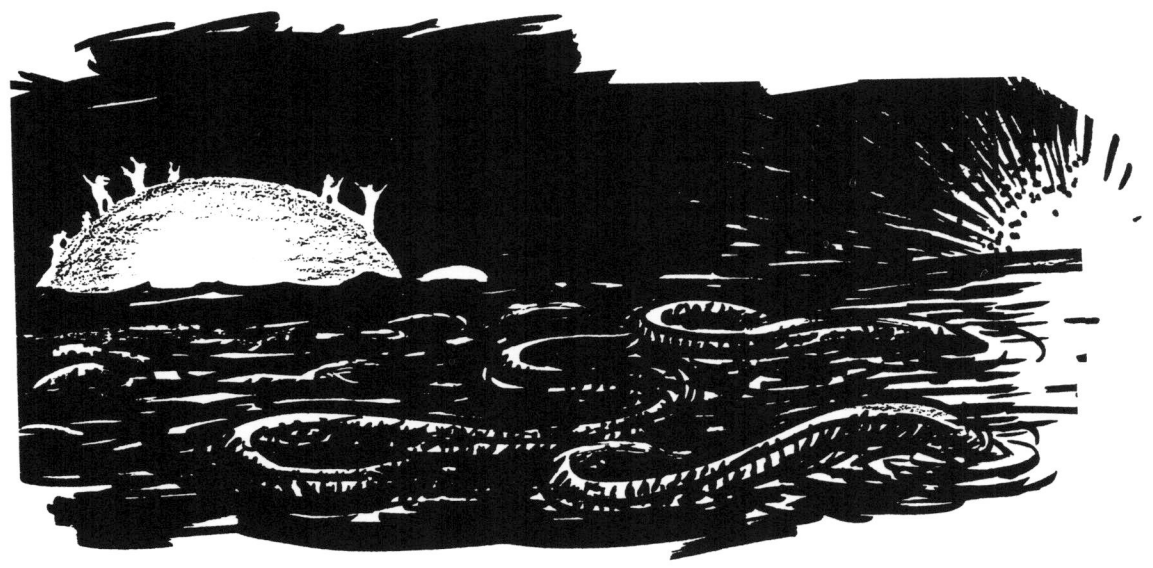

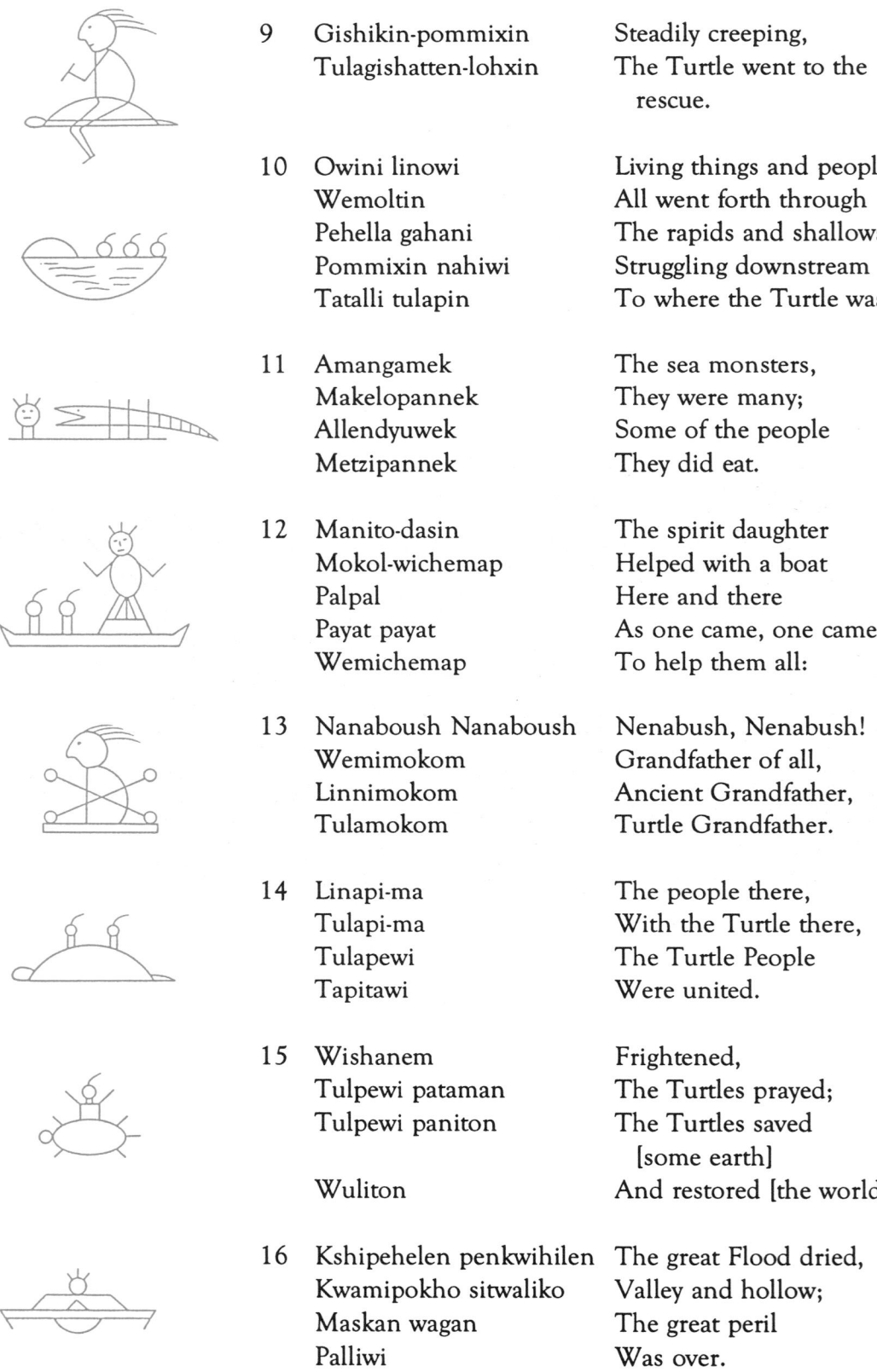

| 9 | Gishikin-pommixin | Steadily creeping, |
| | Tulagishatten-lohxin | The Turtle went to the rescue. |

10	Owini linowi	Living things and people
	Wemoltin	All went forth through
	Pehella gahani	The rapids and shallows,
	Pommixin nahiwi	Struggling downstream
	Tatalli tulapin	To where the Turtle was.

11	Amangamek	The sea monsters,
	Makelopannek	They were many;
	Allendyuwek	Some of the people
	Metzipannek	They did eat.

12	Manito-dasin	The spirit daughter
	Mokol-wichemap	Helped with a boat
	Palpal	Here and there
	Payat payat	As one came, one came
	Wemichemap	To help them all:

13	Nanaboush Nanaboush	Nenabush, Nenabush!
	Wemimokom	Grandfather of all,
	Linnimokom	Ancient Grandfather,
	Tulamokom	Turtle Grandfather.

14	Linapi-ma	The people there,
	Tulapi-ma	With the Turtle there,
	Tulapewi	The Turtle People
	Tapitawi	Were united.

15	Wishanem	Frightened,
	Tulpewi pataman	The Turtles prayed;
	Tulpewi paniton	The Turtles saved [some earth]
	Wuliton	And restored [the world].

16	Kshipehelen penkwihilen	The great Flood dried,
	Kwamipokho sitwaliko	Valley and hollow;
	Maskan wagan	The great peril
	Palliwi	Was over.
	Palliwi	It was over.

The Rescue

Book II: verses 9 through 16

Here we have a continuation of the well-known ancient Native American account of the Flood. Nenabush on the Turtle came to the rescue (II:9) of the people and living things as they battled their way through the surging water (II:10) and the devouring monsters (II:11). Helped by the spirit daughter in her boat (II:12), the people were saved by Nenabush, the great Grandfather (II:13). The addition of the spirit daughter, perhaps the daughter of Nenabush, is an unusual element. She may represent the future destiny of the Lenape people; one reason for the valued position of women in Lenape society is that they represented future generations.

The survivors were united as the Turtle People (II:14). The wording, although obscure, implies a spiritual union with each other, with the Turtle, and, presumably, with Nenabush, who thereafter disappears from the symbols. This may represent the foundation of the oldest Lenni Lenape clan, the Turtle clan.

These Turtle People were frightened and prayed together. They recovered a piece of earth, and from it the world was restored (II:15). The addition of these elements in the translation reflects their almost universal inclusion in the Lenape stories of the Flood. In these stories, the remaking of the world on the back of the Turtle is accomplished with mud brought up by a diving creature.[10] From the hills of this new world to the hollows, the Flood ran off, and the danger pressed far, far away (II:16). (Compare the symbol for this re-created world with the symbol for the first world in I:8.)

Book III

Symbols		Original Words	Translation
	1	Pehellawtenk	After the Flood,
		Lennapewi	The Lenape, the True Men,
		Tulapewini	The Turtle People,
		Psakwiken	Were crowded together,
		Woliwikgun wittanktalli	Living there in cave shelters.
	2	Topan-akpinep	Their home was icy.
		Wineu-akpinep	Their home was snowy.
		Kshakan-akpinep	Their home was windy.
		Thupin-akpinep	Their home was freezing.
	3	Lowankwamink	To the north slope,
		Wulaton	To have
		Wtakan tihill	Less cold,
		Kelik meshautang	Many big-game
		Siliewak	Herds went.
	4	Chitanes-sin	To be strong,
		Powalessin	To be rich;
		Peyachik	The travelers [from]
		Wikhichik	The builders,
		Elowichik	The Hunters
		Pokwihil	Broke away.
	5	Eluwi-chitanesit	Strongest of all,
		Eluwi-takauwesit	Best of all,
		Eluwi-chikset	Holiest of all,
		Elowichik delsinewo	The Hunters are.
	6	Lowaniwi	Northern,
		Wapaniwi	Eastern,
		Shawaniwi	Southern,
		Wunkeniwi	Western;
		Elowichik	The Hunters,
		Apakichik	The Explorers.

A New Beginning

Book III: verses 1 through 6

Book III takes place after the Flood. In its descriptions of distant events, we find the first hints of historical descriptions and indications of a migration beginning from a point deep within Asia.

The Red Record tells how the survivors of the Flood—the Turtle People, the ancestors of the Lenape—lived huddled together in caves (III:1), enduring great cold with harsh weather, storms, and snow (III:2). But to the north, it was milder, and this was where the herds of big-game animals migrated (III:3). Boldly breaking away to follow them, to live well and be blessed (III:4), the best and the bravest, the Hunters (III:5), set out, traveling and exploring in every direction (III:6).

A location for these events is suggested by a reconstruction of the later migration route, which places this, the starting point, in Asia, somewhere along the border between present-day China, Mongolia, and Russia. The descriptions of cave shelters in III:1 and a time of extreme cold in III:2 hint at great antiquity, possibly even as far back as the last Ice Age.

During that time, Western Siberia was heavily glaciated, while Eastern Siberia and Central Asia were almost ice-free. Rainfall increased in every desert area.[11] China was much warmer and wetter than today, with giant turtles crawling through the jungles along the Yangtze.[12] To the north was a challenging but rewarding environment: the glacial steppes around what is now the Gobi Desert, a cold, lush grassland, where dry, dust-laden winds swirled, and where great herds of large migrating herbivores grazed, as suggested in III:3.[13] New forms of stone points enabled daring hunters to slay even these massive beasts, making possible a life following the herds.

Around 6000 B.C., as the hunters followed the herds into the north, the first settled farming communities began to appear to the south along the Hwang Ho River.[14] In the symbol for III:4, the figure on the left seems to be the settler, and may be holding a hoe, while the other figure may be holding aloft an important invention for hunting, the atlatl or spear-thrower. In III:5, the Hunter is shown holding in the right hand a barbed and feathered arrow for a bow, a more recent invention. The other hand may hold a medicine bag, a game animal or its skin, or even a paddle for a canoe. These hunters or explorers moved out in every direction. The recitation of the directions in III:6 is clockwise; throughout the Red Record, compound symbols are always read in a clockwise order.

By 3000 B.C., the glaciers and the massive Ice Age animals had vanished, but the hunters of the North continued to adapt and prosper. Excavations at a cave on the Shilka River near the Amur illuminate the way of life that then extended from Lake Baikal to the Amur and into the north. The people had dogs, made pottery, used arrows and fishing tackle, and probably also had boats for river travel.[15]

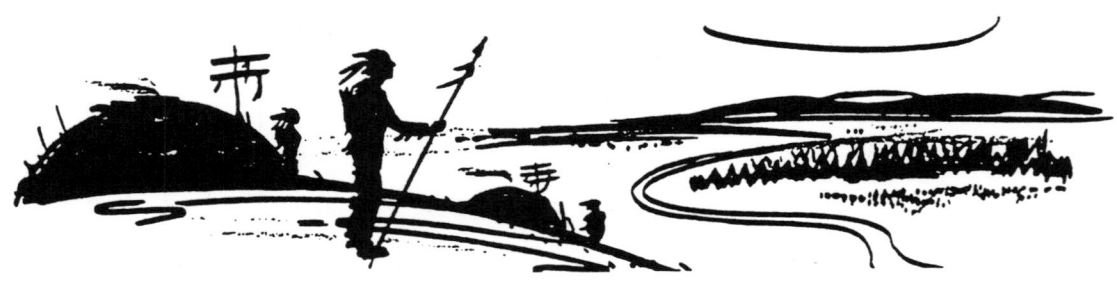

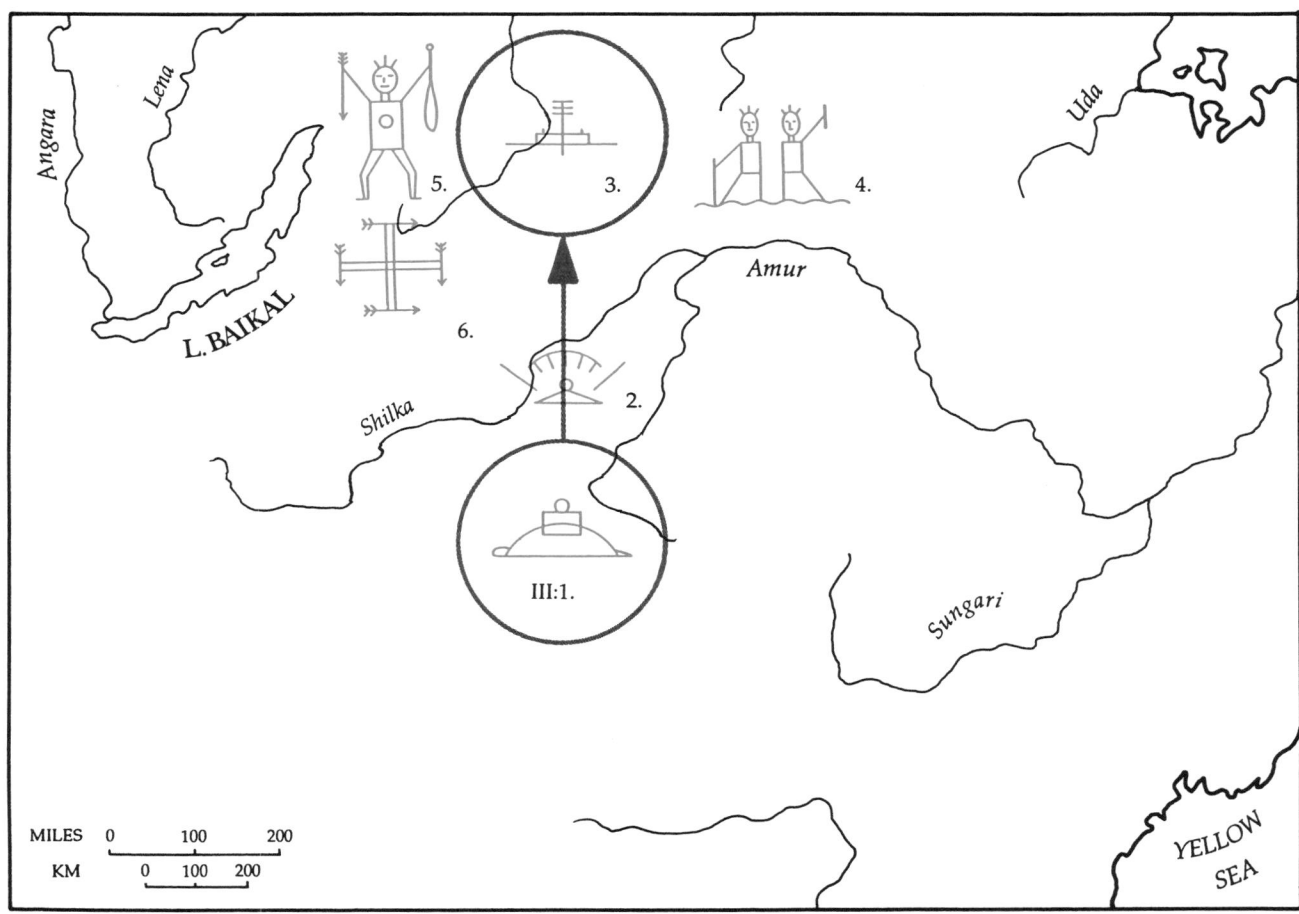

Figure 4.2. The map shows the migration route as revealed in verses 1 through 6 of Book III. The numbers on the map and in the box below refer to the verses in which the symbols and location clues appear.

Location Clues

1. Locations for this earliest part of the story are very approximate. A systematic plotting of the migration route places this, the starting point, near where the borders of present-day Russia, China, and Mongolia meet.

2. The symbol shows wind and snow threatening the Lenape; such harsh weather is characteristic of this rugged and barren border region.

3. The Lenape cross into Siberia, into a northward-flowing watershed.

4. The settled agrarian culture of China lies to the south; beyond the Amur, survival depends on travel and hunting. Note the river symbol connecting the figures in this verse. (This is a generalized location, which means that the symbol refers to an overall region rather than to a specific place.)

5. Heroic hunters are valued in native cultures both in Asia and America. (This, too, is a general location.)

6. The region of Lake Baikal ("Lake of the Spirits") is the meeting place of watersheds that flow to the north, east, and west (general location).

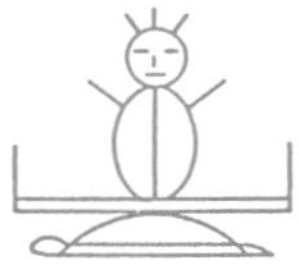

7 Lumowaki lowanaki

In the old land, the
winter land,

Tulpenaki elowaki

The Turtle land, the
great land,

Tulapewi linapiwi

Were the Turtle Men,
the Lenape.

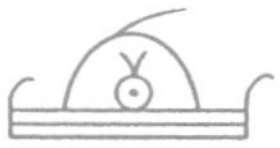

8 Wemiako
Yagawan tendki
Lakkawelendam
    nakopowa
Wemiowenluen atam

All the enemy Snake
Lodge fires
Were troubled; the Snake
   priest
Said to them all, "Let us go."

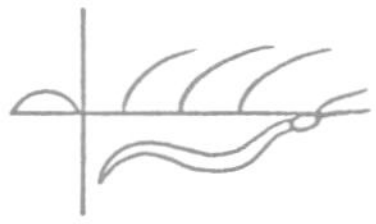

9 Akhokink wapaneu

The Snakes there in the
east

Wemoltin palliaal
Kitelendam aptelendam

All went forth, going away,
Grim, and grieving.

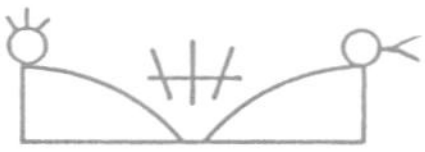

10 Pechimuin
Shakowen nungihillan
Lusasaki
Pikihil Pokwihil
Akomenaki

Fleeing,
Tired and shivering,
Through the wasteland;
Torn and broken,
To Akomen, the
   Wilderness.

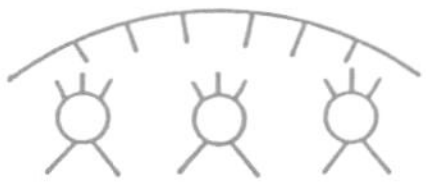

11 Nihillapewin
Komelendam
Lowaniwi wemiten
Chihillen
Winiaken

The free men,
Carefree and fearless,
All went northward,
Spreading across
The snowy country.

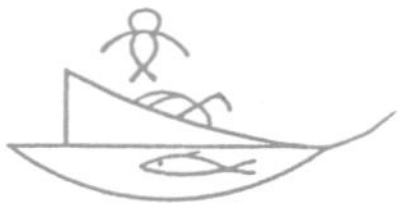

12 Namesuagipek
Pokhapokhapek
Guneunga Waplanewa
    ouken
Waptumewi ouken

By the dark fish sea,
The gaping hollow sea,
Settled the White Eagle
   clan and
The White Wolf clan.

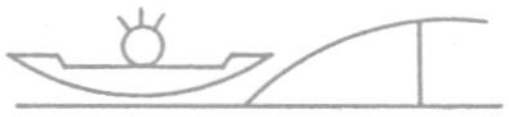

13 Amokolen nallahemen
Agunouken pawasinep
Wapasinep
Akomenep

Rowing, crossing the water,
For long they gloried
In the eastern light,
In the land of Akomen.

The Enemy Withdraws

Book III: verses 7 through 13

In the North, the best land, were the Turtle People, the Lenape (III:7). To the east were the Snake enemies. Seen from the Lenape point of view, all enemies were Snakes, and included those in the south as well as those in the east. A glimpse of the ancestors of the Lenape may have been preserved by their enemies to the south, the Chinese.

From its earliest days, China has struggled with the restless tribes of Mongolia and beyond, a conflict that eventually led to the construction of the Great Wall. The war between the Turtle People of the north and the Snake (or Dragon) people of the south who later became the Chinese is told in ancient histories by the earliest Chinese historians. Among the earliest mentioned were the Hiung-nu, who were driven away by Huang-ti, the "Yellow Emperor," around 2600 B.C.[16] It is recorded that the Turtle People eventually vanished into the far north. In Chinese tradition, the turtle is still the symbol for the North. Since turtles are not found in northern climates, the symbol may be based on a memory of a northern antagonist such as the Lenape, who called themselves the Turtle People. The possibility of contact between the proto-Chinese and a large population that later crossed over into America has been supported by evidence of Chinese influence dating from the time of the Shang Dynasty. This influence on an Eskimo population has been revealed by the Ipiutak excavations in Alaska.[17]

The Snake enemies scattered (III:8), fleeing eastward across the wastelands (III:9) and crossing into the land of Akomen (III:10). "Akomen," the ancient name for the unknown land that became the New World, is usually translated as "Snake Island," but it also connotes "The Wilderness" and "The Land Beyond."

The bold and fearless Lenape spread across the snowy country to the north (III:11). A reconstruction of their route indicates that at this point, they would have been entering the coldest place in the northern hemisphere. Northeastern Siberia even today is a vast and forbidding region of bare mountains and windswept tundra. In the wake of the Ice Age, it was a brutal environment, an arctic desert tormented by fierce storms. But along its eastern edge by the Bering Sea was a marine environment that was full of life—including whales, seals, and walrus—and could support a permanent population.[18]

The Red Record describes how the White Wolf clan and the White Eagle clan settled by an ocean channel (III:12). The descriptions of this channel in III:12 and in III:17 strongly suggest the Bering Strait. Note that no mention is made of a land bridge.

Rowing across the water into Akomen, explorers from the Wolf and White Eagle clans found a land of richness and promise (III:13). The Yukon valley beyond the Bering Strait in Alaska remained relatively green and ice-free, even during the Ice Age, and was, therefore, an attractive place for migrating birds. White Eagle is later identified in IV:2 as the leader in the movement to the New World. The words in III:13 imply that Akomen was a "land of their dreams."

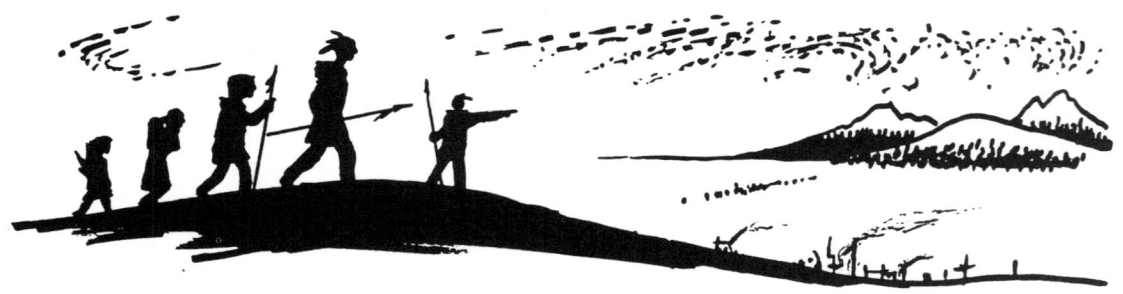

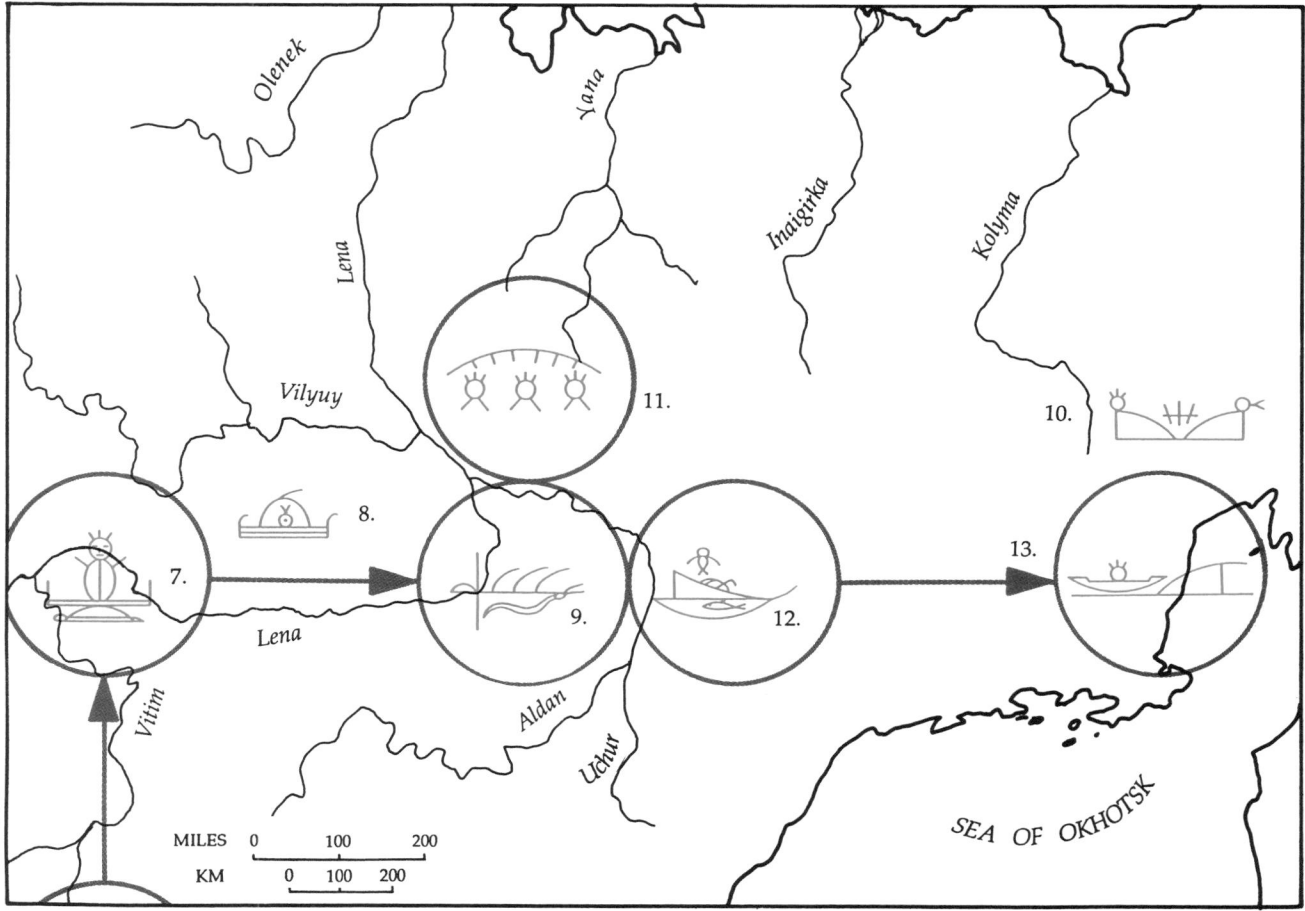

Figure 4.3. The map shows the migration route as revealed in verses 7 through 13 of Book III. The numbers on the map and in the box below refer to the verses in which the symbols and location clues appear.

Location Clues

7. Here, the Lenape are along the middle of the Lena River, the greatest river of central Siberia.

8. The rounded shape of the snake lodge in this symbol is characteristic of ancient semi-subterranean Siberian houses.

9, 10. Any journey across the mountains of northeastern Siberia is extremely difficult even today. Only the strongest can survive. The symbol indicates a crossing from one continent to another and refers to an overall region rather than a specific place (general location).

11. The words and symbols indicate movement into a part of Siberia that is the coldest region on Earth outside of Antarctica.

12. Another indicated movement takes a portion of the Lenape to the shoreline, to the maritime environment of the Sea of Okhotsk and the Bering Sea across the Kamchatka Peninsula to the east. "White Eagle" could refer to the bald eagle or the fish-eating hawk called the osprey; "White Wolf" could refer to the winter appearance of the Arctic fox.

13. The words and symbol clearly indicate an exploration of Alaska, probably by an ascent of the Yukon River (general location).

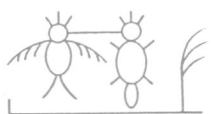

14 Wihlamok   Beaver Head and
     Kicholen   Great Bird,
     Luchundi wematam   They said, "Let us go!"
     Akomen luchundi   "To Akomen!" they said.

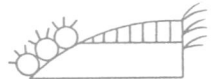

15 Witehen   The allies
     Wemiluen   All declared,
     Wemaken   "All our enemies
     Nihillen   Will be destroyed."

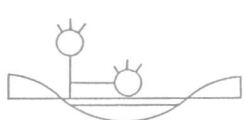

16 Nguttichin lowaniwi   The northerners agreed,
     Nguttichin wapaniwi   The easterners agreed,
     Agamunk topanpek   Across the icy ocean
     Wulliton epannek   Was a better place to be.

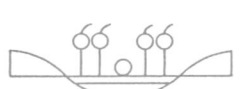

17 Wulelemil w'shakuppek   On a wondrous sheet of ice
     Wemopannek   All crossed the frozen sea
         hakhsinipek
     Kitahikan   At low tide in the
     Pokhakhopek   Narrows of the ocean.

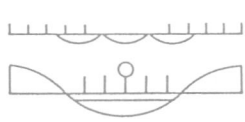

18 Tellenchen kittapakki   Ten times a thousand,
     Nillawi   They crossed;
     Wemoltin gutikuni   All went forth in a night;
     Nillawi   They crossed
     Akomen wapanaki   To Akomen, the East Land,
         nillawi   crossing,
     Ponskan ponskan   Marching, marching,
     Wemiwi olini   Everyone together.

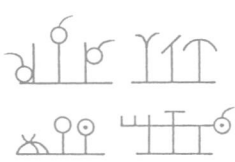

19 Lowanapi wapanapi   People of the North, the East,
     Shawanapi lanewapi   The South; of the Eagle,
     Tamakwapi tumewapi   Of the Beaver, of the Wolf;
     Elowapi powatapi   The Hunters, Shamans,
         wilawapi   Headmen;
     Okwisapi danisapi   The Women, Daughters,
         allumapi   Animals;

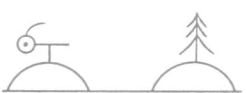

20 Wemipayat gunéunga   All came to settle
     Shinaking   In the evergreen land.
     Wunkenapi chanelendam   The western people reluctantly
     Payaking allowelendam   Came there, for they loved it best
     Kowiyey-tulpaking   In the old Turtle country.

The Crossing to the New World

Book III: verses 14 through 20

The news of the better land across the ocean was enough to convince Wihlamok (Beaver Head) and Kicholen (Great Bird) to urge all the Lenape clans to unite to cross the sea into the New World (III:14). There they would win a better land and a better life from their enemies (III:15–16). Wihlamok and Kicholen may be historical figures or the name of a clan.

Ten thousand strong, the Lenape crossed the frozen sea to the evergreen country (III:17–19). Only those from the West preferred to remain where they had been (III:14). The earlier reference to the eastern Snakes who crossed over first into the New World (III:10) is a clear statement that when the Lenape reached North America it was already inhabited. That this verse refers to a crossing of the Bering Strait from Asia to America is supported not only by a reconstruction of the route described in the Red Record, but also by other accounts from the Lenni Lenape and their nearest relatives (see page 38).

Given careful planning and preparation, it is possible that ten thousand could cross in a year or less. The words in III:18 say "in a night," but this probably means "in one dark season," referring to the winter, the most likely time for the Bering Strait to freeze over as described here.

A representation of the quantity "ten thousand" in the top part of the symbol for III:18 would be unique, as there are no other indications of large numbers in the Red Record. Although the Lenni Lenape had a method of counting to ten thousand,[19] it is possible that this symbol may represent something else, such as a passage over a total of three bodies of water.

The symbols of the clans, geographical groups, and social classes among the Lenape in III:19 is also unique; as a listing of the components of ancient Lenape society, it is of great anthropological interest. These four groups of symbols are read clockwise, starting with the group at the upper left. Within each group of three, the center element is apparently read first, then the right, then the left. This verse contains the first written record of any Native American group's crossing of the Bering Strait from Asia to America. However, there is nothing to suggest that there may not have been other crossings in the other direction, from America to Asia.

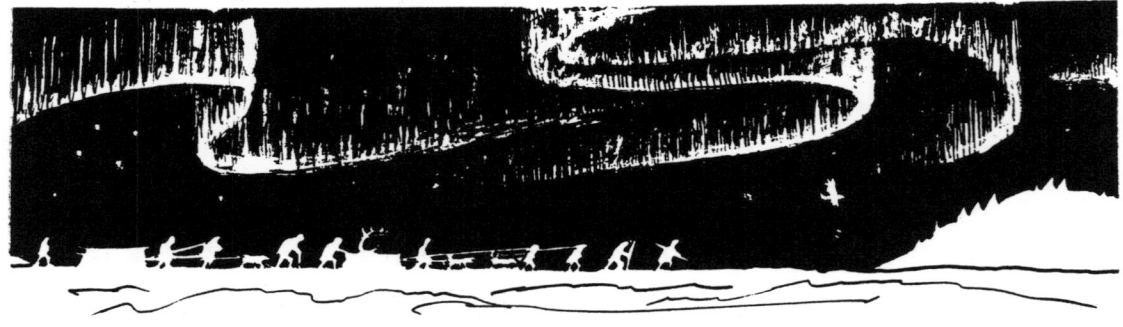

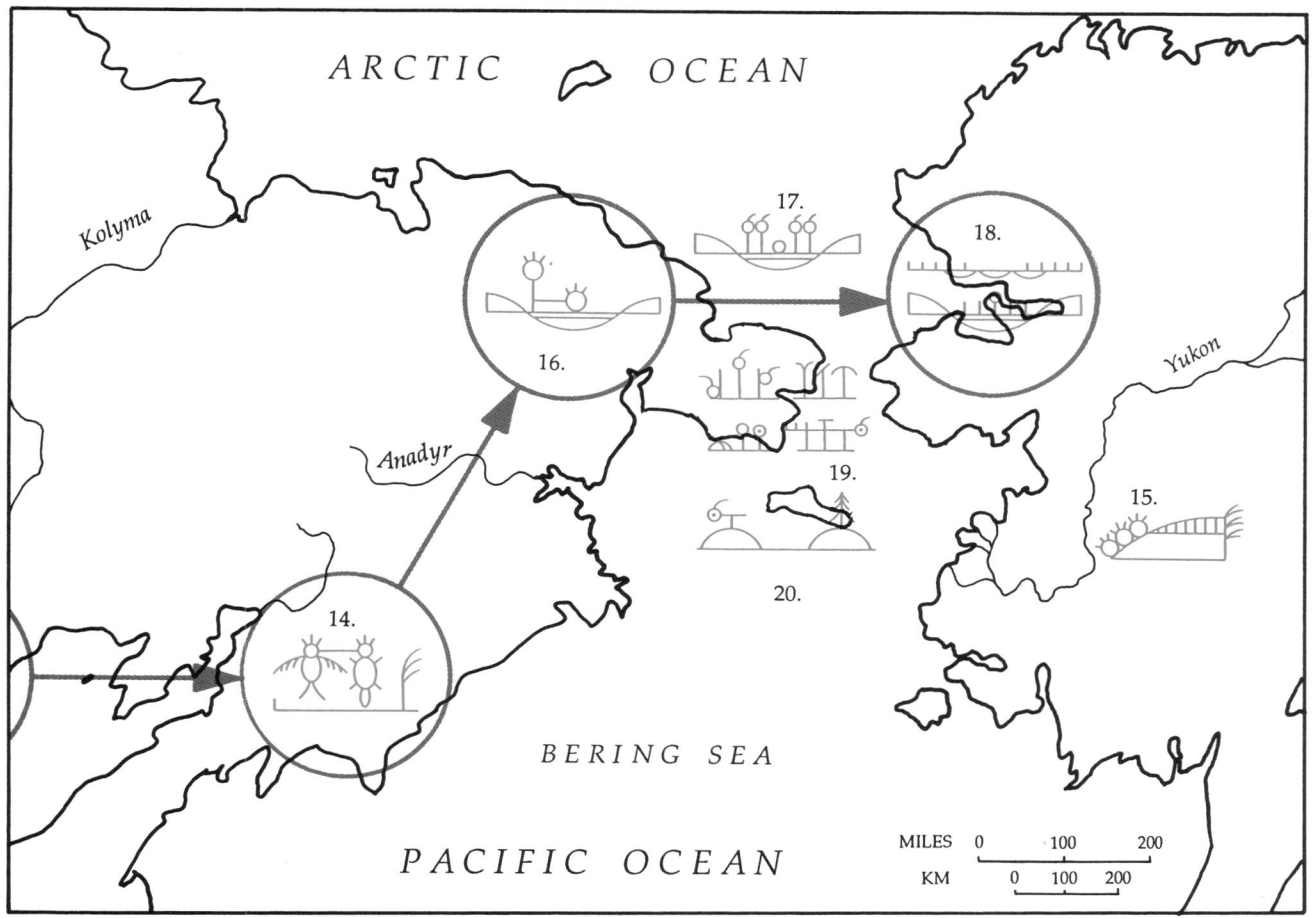

Figure 4.4. The map shows the migration route as revealed in verses 14 through 20 of Book III. The numbers on the map and in the box below refer to the verses in which the symbols and location clues appear.

Location Clues

14. The indicated movement takes the Lenape to the shores of the Bering Sea.

15. The symbol indicates a planned invasion of Akomen, where the enemy is shown as occupying the interior (general location).

16. The northeastern Lenape are the leaders in the movement to the New World. The symbol indicates the ocean passage between the continents and the ice bridge.

17. The Lenape are represented crossing the ice.

18. The pairs of vertical lines on either side of the figure could indicate the hardship of the crossing (see IV:27, IV:56).

19. The "Animals" in this verse could be dogs for dogsleds.

20. The symbol represents the eastern and western continents or "Turtle Islands," with the forests of Alaska indicated (general location).

Book IV

Symbols	**Original Words**	**Translation**
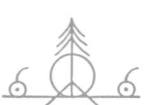	1 Wulamo Linapioken Manup Shinaking	Long ago, The ancient Lenape Came to The evergreen land.
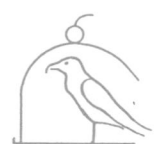	2 Wapallanewa Sittamaganat Yukepechi Wemima	The White Eagle Had been the path-maker Hitherto For all of them there.
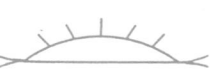	3 Akhomenis Michihaki Wellaki Kundokanup	When Akomen, The ready land, The good land, They discovered.
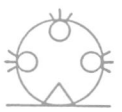	4 Angomelchik Elowichik Elmusichik Menalting	The kindred, The Hunters, The pioneers Meeting in council,
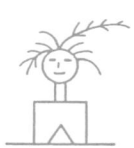	5 Wemilo Kolawil Sakima Lissilma	All declared, "Kolawil, Noble Elder, Thou art sachem Here."
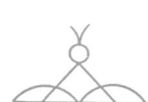	6 Akhopayat Kihillalend Akhopokho Askiwaal	"The Snakes come; Thou must slay them; The Snake hollow They must leave."
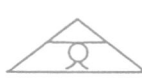	7 Showihilla Akhowemi Gandhaton Mashkipokhing	Defeated, All the Snakes Fled to hide In the swampy vales.
	8 Wtenkolawil Shinaking Sakimanep Wapagokhos	After Kolawil In the evergreen land The sachem was The White Owl.

Leaders in the Forest

Book IV: verses 1 through 8

Book IV begins with a description of the Lenape in a new forest home (IV:1), which probably represents the Yukon River valley. Wapallanewa, the White Eagle, was the visonary explorer who had led them to this new world they called Akomen (IV:3). Wapallanewa may be an individual and may be connected to the White Eagle clan mentioned earlier in III:12. The name of this first recorded discoverer of America refers to the bald eagle, the national symbol of the United States.

Having followed White Eagle, the Lenape now faced a challenge from their enemies in the new land, the Snakes, and needed a new kind of leader to lead them into battle. The Lenape clans gathered together in council (IV:4), and elected Kolawil, the Noble Elder (IV:5), to be their sachem or chief.

Kolawil appears to have been primarily a war leader, one who could command obedience. Peacetime leaders ruled solely through persuasion.[20] The election of Kolawil as sachem marks the beginning of a succession of ninety-six leaders listed in the Red Record, a succession that can be continued through the Fragment included in the Rafinesque Manuscript and other historical records up to the present day. This is the longest uninterrupted history of leadership in the New World.

Kolawil led the Lenape warriors against the Snakes (IV:6), and the Lenape were victorious, driving the Snakes away into distant swamps and wastelands (IV:7). Thus, the Snakes were confined to the tundra around the periphery of Alaska, while the Lenape were free to move deeper into the forested interior.

The Lenape moved up the Yukon valley under Kolawil's successor White Owl (IV:8).

This succession may have been through election or through inheritance. Kinship and inheritance customs were complex and differed widely among the Lenape of historical times, so it is difficult to extrapolate to this period. While the Lenni Lenape on the East Coast, as well as some of the interior Alaskan tribes, favored matriarchal descent (through the female line), other tribes in Alaska had no preference, and there were Lenape tribes in the Midwest that favored patriarchal descent.[21] Probably the means of succession, as well as the power of the sachem, varied throughout Lenape history.

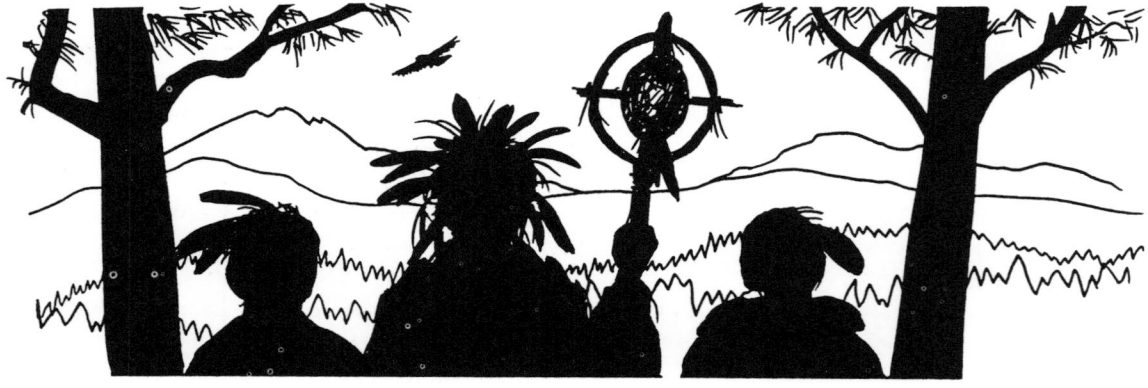

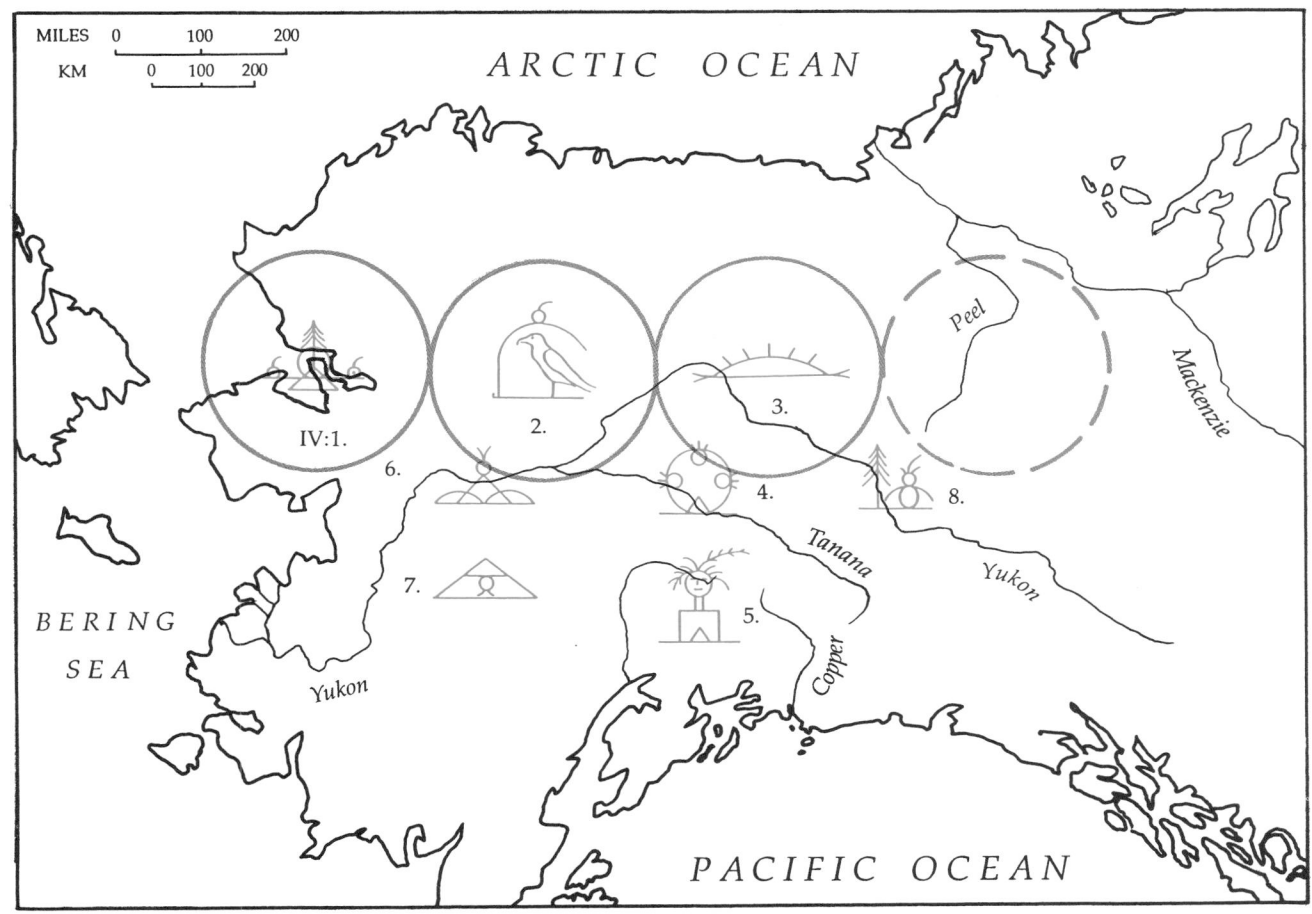

Figure 4.5. The map shows the migration route as revealed in verses 1 through 8 of Book IV. The numbers on the map and in the box below refer to the verses in which the symbols and location clues appear. The broken-line circle indicates that the movement has been inferred by the author rather than directly stated in the words and/or symbols.

Location Clues

1. The Lenape came to Alaska, which is relatively greener than Siberia.

2. The sachem is White Eagle. White animals were generally considered as animal chiefs and were, therefore, sacred; the magnificent, white-headed bald eagle is still a symbol of America.

3. The forks on either side of the symbol indicate occupation by the Snakes.

4, 5. The symbols, which indicate the election of a new sachem and the establishment of a new council fire, refer to an overall region rather than a specific place (general location).

6. The symbol represents the space between hills, and may indicate the Yukon River valley. (This, too, is a general location.)

7. The "swampy vales" suggest the boggy tundra around the shores of Alaska, so the Snakes were apparently driven from the forested interior onto the coastal plain. Even today, there is a marked distinction in appearance and customs between the Native American people of the Alaskan interior and the Eskimo (Inuit) people of the coast (general location).

8. Again, there are clear indications of a forest home. Here, the sachem is White Owl; the snowy owl is a large white owl found in arctic regions.

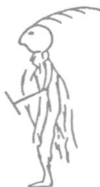

9   Wtenknekama   After him,
    Sakimanep   The sachem was
    Janotowi   Constantly
    Enolowin   On Guard.

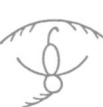

10 Wtenknekama   After him,
    Sakimanep   The sachem was
    Chilili   Chilili, the Snow Bird,
    Shawaniluen   Who spoke of the south.

11 Wokenapi   That our people
    Nitaton   Would be able
    Wullaton   To grow and
    Apakchikton   Spread there.

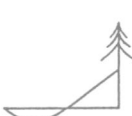

12 Shawaniwaen   Southward went
    Chilili   Chilili;
    Wapaniwaen   Eastward went
    Tamakwi   The Beaver.

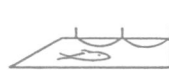

13 Akolaki   To Akolaki, Snake Land,
    Shawanaki   Southern country,
    Kitshinaki   Tall pine country,
    Shabiyaki   Seashore country.

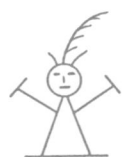

14 Wapanaki   To Eastern country,
    Namesaki   Fishing country,
    Pemapaki   Mountain country,
    Sisilaki   Game herd country.

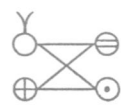

15 Wtenkchilili   After Chilili
    Sakimanep   The sachem was
    Ayamek   Ayamek, The Seizer;
    Weminilluk   He slew them all:

16 Chikonapi   The Charlatans,
    Akhonapi   The Snakes,
    Makatapi   The Blackened Ones,
    Assinapi   The Stony Ones.

Into the East and Along the Shore

Book IV: verses 9 through 16

The Lenape remained on guard against the Snakes (IV:9). Chilili, the Snow Bird, found the land of Akolaki to the south to be a more desirable place (IV:10), and urged the Lenape to spread out and take possession of it (IV:11). (Akolaki is a complex term that suggests both "Snake Land" and "Beautiful Land.") So the Lenape split in two, with Chilili leading half southward into the rich coastland of Akolaki. The rest, led by Beaver, continued eastward, going upstream into the Yukon valley (IV:12–14). In the past, anthropologists assumed that during glacial and postglacial times, tribes migrating southward would have had to follow a route through the mountain valleys inland. But recently, a coastal route down the Northwest Coast, employing boats, has been described as just as desirable.[22] The Lenape seem to have taken both routes, based on a preference for one region or the other.

A Shawnee legend of a long canoe journey leading to the discovery of a rich shoreland may be a reference to Chilili's exploration of the south as related in IV:10. It may, however, be a reference to the earlier explorations of White Eagle and White Wolf recounted in III:12–13.[23]

Life on the Northwest Coast was a life of relative ease and abundance, drawing on the marine life offshore and the regular migrations of salmon inland from the ocean. The tall evergreen woods also yielded the materials for elaborate crafts, boats, and houses. The leisure time afforded by this abundance was often occupied by raiding and warfare, with captives sometimes made into slaves.

The Lenape conquered a new territory under Chilili's successor, Ayamek, The Seizer (IV:15), who slew all of their enemies (IV:16). Ayamek's character is hard to gauge, but there are indications that he may have been greedy and ruthless, for after him there is a time of great evil. There is also a hint of black magic in the identification in IV:16 of two of the enemies as the "Blackened Ones" and the "Charlatans." This recalls the culture of the Northwest Coast, where sorcery and war by magic were prevalent.[24]

It is difficult to determine the present identities of these and other enemy tribes mentioned in the Red Record, since the Lenape tended to use "snake" as a generic term for "enemy." But if the Red Record's symbols refer to language differences, later clues in the symbols, the story, and other historical records suggest that the Stony Ones may be from the Siouan or the Shoshonean language family, while the Snakes may be from the Siouan language family. The other tribes mentioned here may refer to people from the Na-Dene language group, such as the Tlingit and Haida, who can be found on the Northwest Coast today.

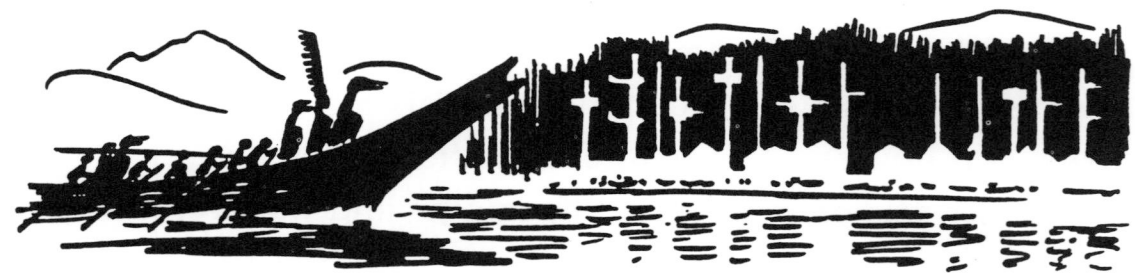

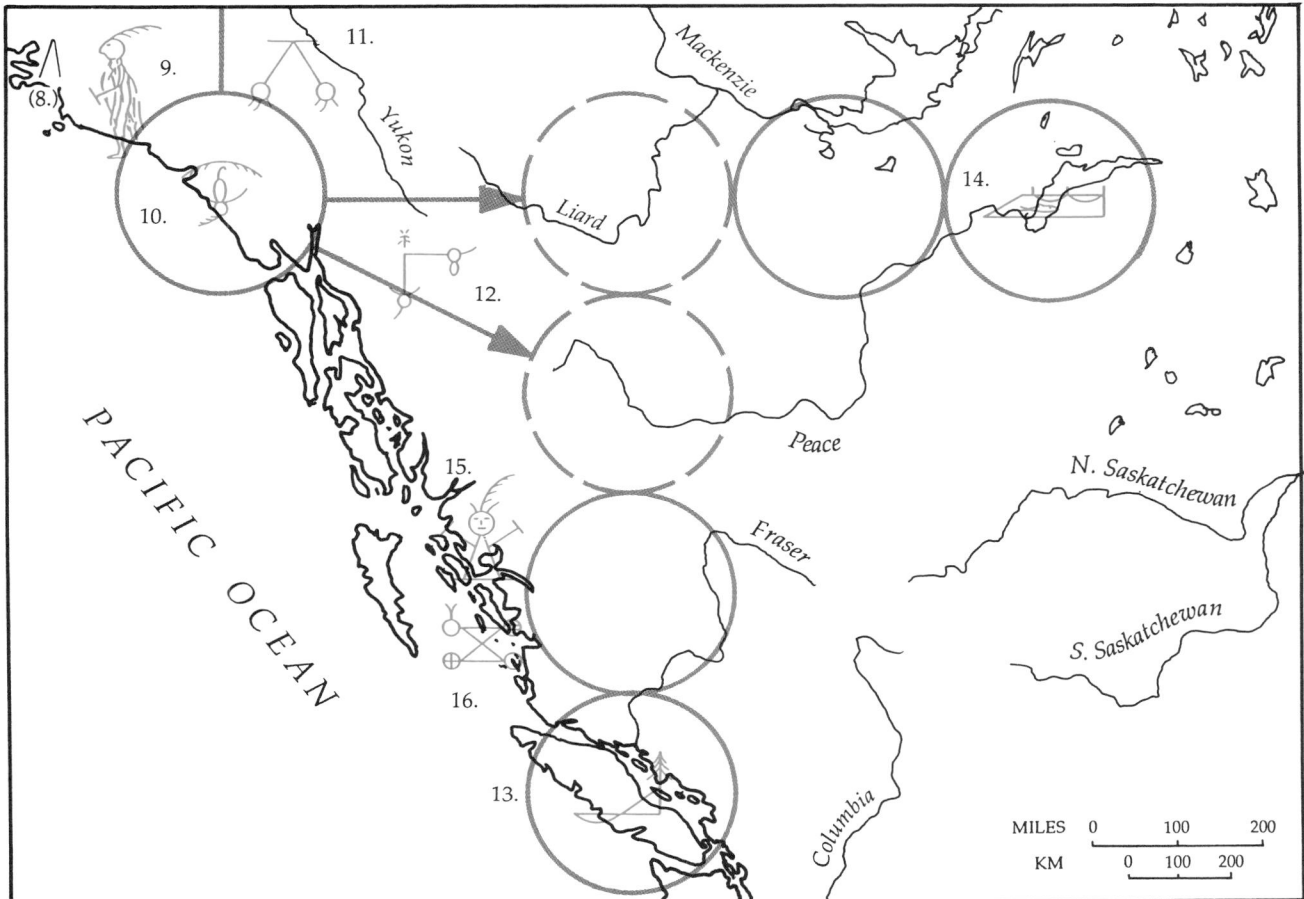

Figure 4.6. The map shows the migration route as revealed in verses **9** through **16** of Book IV. The numbers on the map and in the box below refer to the verses in which the symbols and location clues appear. Broken-line circles indicate that the movement has been inferred by the author rather than directly stated in the words and/or symbols.

Location Clues

9. At this time, the Lenape were located in the Yukon valley in Alaska.

10. The name "Snow Bird" may reflect the high mountains and glaciers that separate Alaska from the Pacific rain forest and the rich maritime environment of the Northwest Coast.

11. The words and symbol indicate a planned division into more than one territory.

12. To the south is the Northwest Coast; inland, the rivers flow eastward beyond the Rockies into a vast region of boreal forests.

13. The region called Akolaki in this verse is more commonly known as the Northwest Coast, a heavily forested land of great natural abundance.

14. To the east, the Canadian Rockies gradually give way to a vast plain with innumerable lakes and streams.

15. In this verse, the sachem "slew them all." The Northwest Coast in historic times was known for its wars.

16. A wide variety of tribal groups occupied the maze of islands and waterways of the Northwest Coast.

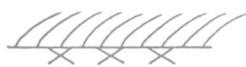

17	Wtenkayamek Tellensakimak Machitonanup Shawapama	After Ayamek, Ten sachems; Much evil was then South and eastward.

18	Wtenknellamawa Sakimanep Langundowi Akolaking	After them, The sachem was The Peaceful One In Akolaki.

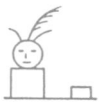

19	Wtenknekama Sakimanep Tasukamend Shakagapewi	After him, The sachem was The Blameless One, Honest and Upright.

20	Wtenknekama Sakimanep Pemoholend Wulitowin	After him, The sachem was Constant Love, Who brought goodness.

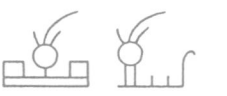

21	Sakimawtenk Matemik Sakimawtenk Pilsohalin	The next sachem was House Maker; The next sachem was Chastely Loving.

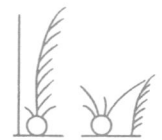

22	Sakimawtenk Gunokeni Sakimawtenk Mangipitak	The next sachem was Long Lineage; The next sachem was Big Teeth.

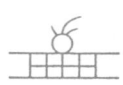

23	Sakimawtenk Olumapi Leksahowen Sohalawak	The next sachem was History Man; Written records He began.

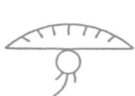

24	Sakimawtenk Taquachi Shawaniwaen Minihaking	The next sachem was Frozen One, Who went southward To the fruitful fields.

Corruption and Rebirth

Book IV: verses 17 through 24

There was a time of great war and evil (IV:17). The ten chiefs associated with these evil events are the only ones in the Red Record not mentioned by name. Omitting the names may be connected with the Delaware belief that bad people deserve to be forgotten, while the good deserve to live on in memory. This belief is a powerful incentive for keeping chronicles, such as the Red Record, of past heroes.

The nature of these evil events is also not specified, but there are clues provided by the names of the subsequent sachems. Apparently in reaction to the unknown evil, the later sachems were first Peaceful One (IV:18), then Blameless One, "Honest and Upright" (IV:19). Then came Constant Love, House Maker, and Chastely Loving (IV:20–21). The opposite of these virtues may be some of the unnamed vices that dominated the evil time: wrath and violence, greed and corruption, betrayal, laziness, and lechery.

Two of the most ancient religious features of the Lenni Lenape, the Big House Ceremony and the Mising Mask, may have had their origins at this time. Delaware legend says they were learned after a time of evil and impiety, following a severe punishment described as including a full year of earthquakes (earthquakes are a well-known feature of the coast of Alaska).[25]

Peaceful One is specified as being in Akolaki, but that portion of the Lenape who, in IV:12, had gone inland under Beaver is not identified again. The group may have vanished from the story into the east, perhaps to become the ancestors of such

Canadian tribes as the Cree. However, the group may have rejoined the main body in the vicinity of Akolaki in an unidentified reunion, perhaps indicated by the dualities in the symbols for IV:19, IV:21, and IV:22.

Following this period, Olumapi (History Man) invented a method of record-keeping to help preserve Lenape history and Lenape geneology (IV:23). Olumapi is the thirteenth named sachem (the twenty-third sachem if the unnamed ten in IV:17 are counted), and is credited with the invention of written records. (Anthropological studies suggest that purely oral traditions begin to break down after a certain number of generations unless some form of symbol-writing is invented to aid the memory.) It is interesting that the symbol for Olumapi in IV:23 resembles the Chinese pictogram for "book," which depicts bamboo slats tied together side to side with cords, the writing surface used before the invention of paper.[26]

The sachem after Olumapi was Frozen One. During his time, the Lenape moved southward to a warmer and more fruitful country (IV:24) in the region of the Great Plateau.

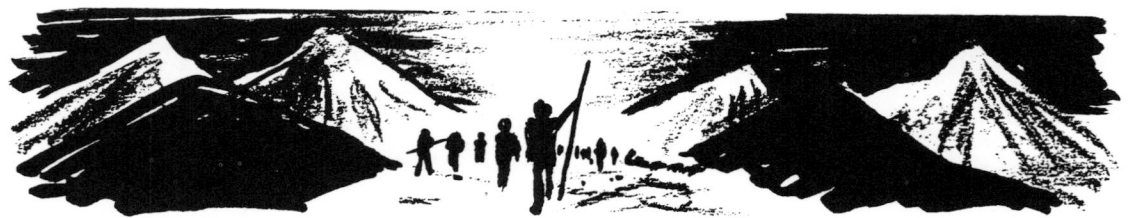

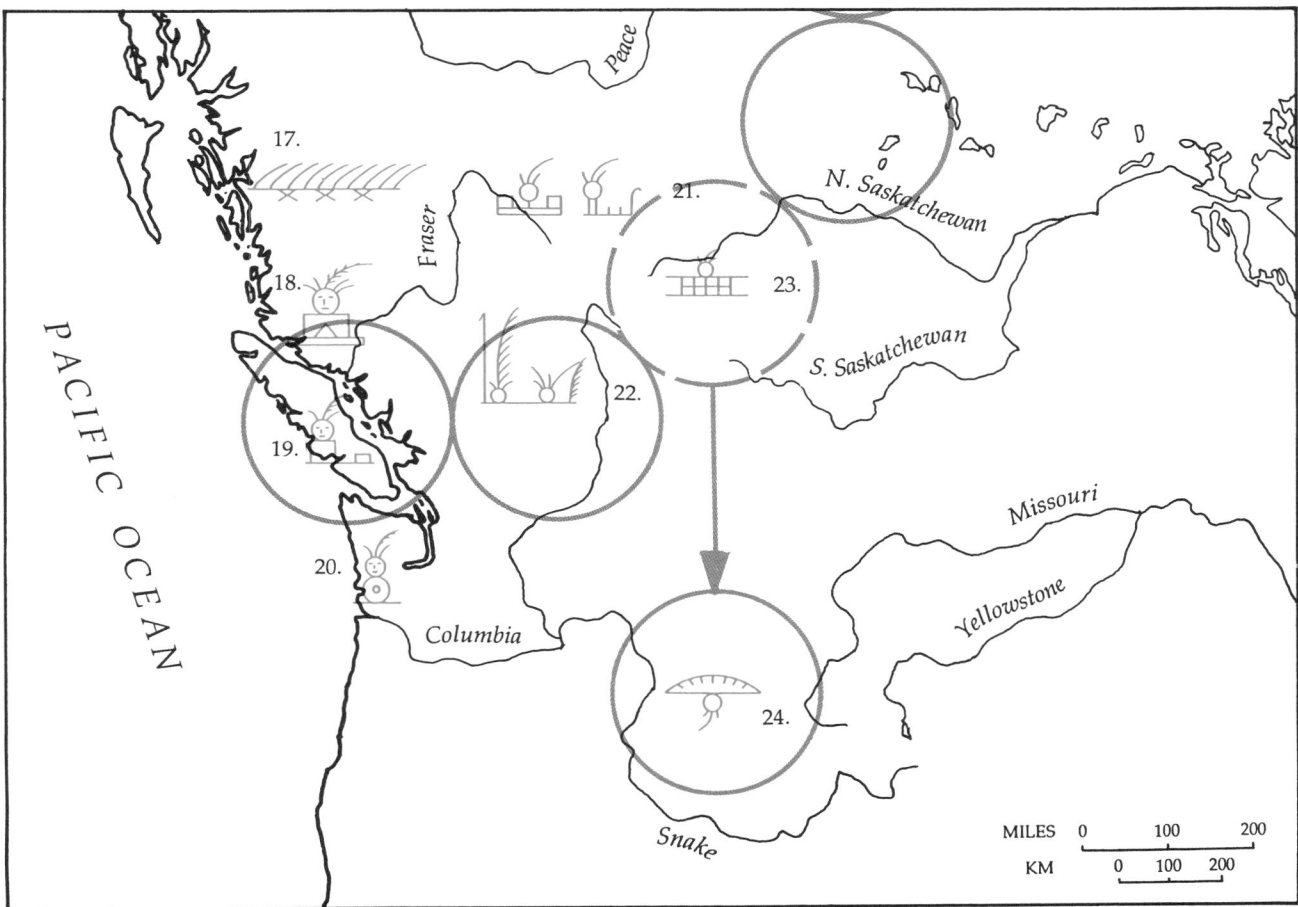

Figure 4.7. The map shows the migration route as revealed in verses **17** through **24** of **Book IV**. The numbers on the map and in the box below refer to the verses in which the symbols and location clues appear. The broken-line circle indicates that the movement has been inferred by the author rather than directly stated in the words and/or symbols.

Location Clues

17. The evil events appear to be primarily in Akolaki.

18, 19. Both verses seem to be related to Akolaki, although the small rectangle in the second symbol may refer to the Lenape in the east.

20, 21. This dual symbol contains references to the two branches of the Lenape: the symbol for House Maker indicates a powerful chief in a territory between two establishments, while the symbol for Chastely Loving suggests some difficulty (the short vertical lines) between the chief and the curved line pointing toward the east.

22. In this dual symbol, a contrast may be implied between the Lenape in the west (Long Lineage) and the chief in the east (Big Teeth), who seems to have broken symbols of memory and authority.

23. This verse, which mentions History Man and the invention of written records, seems to refer to the reunion of the Lenape and a formalization of their traditions. The location is, therefore, placed midway between the locations of the two divisions.

24. This verse reflects the change of climate and diet found as one enters the Great Plateau from the north.

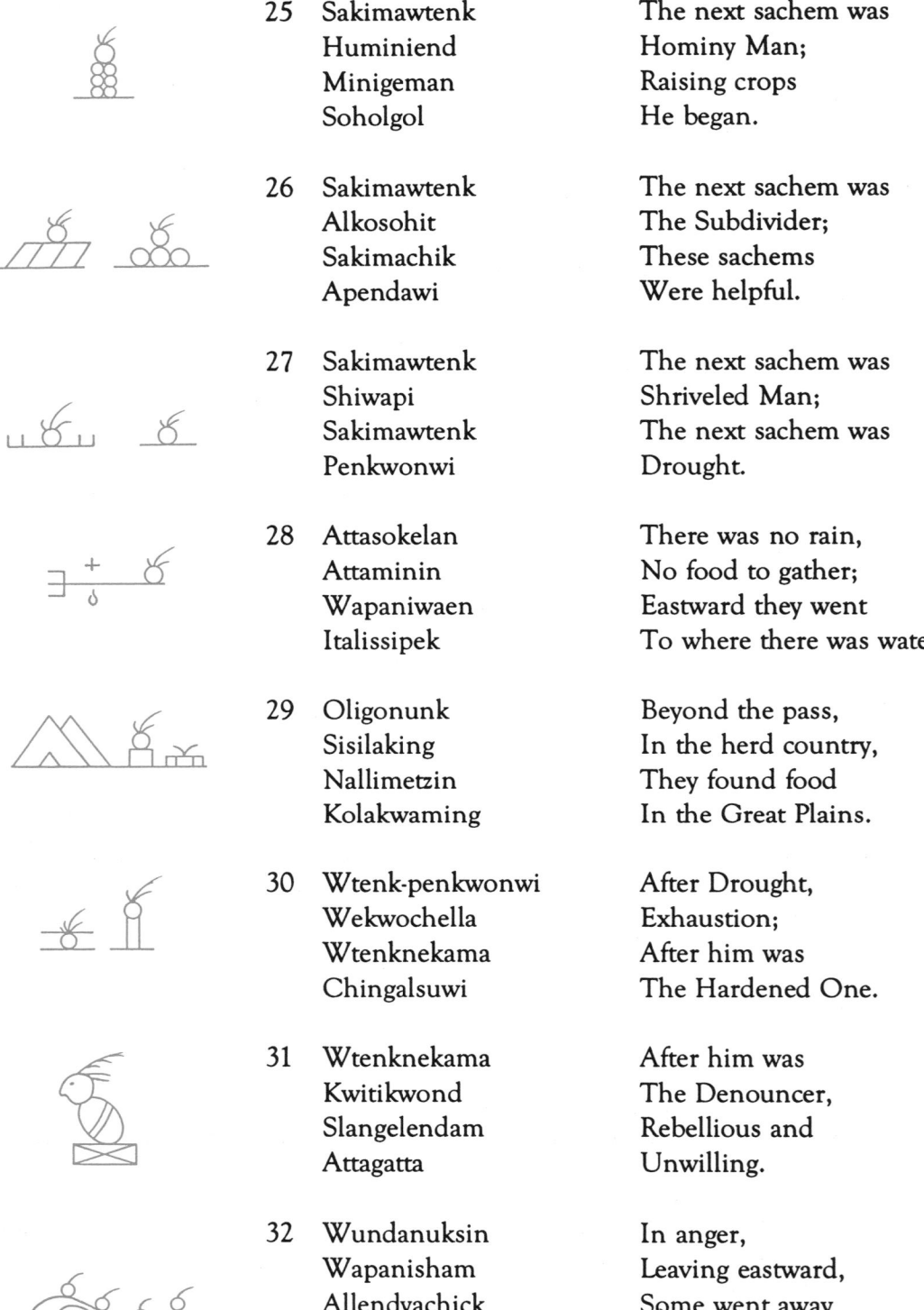

25 Sakimawtenk   The next sachem was
   Huminiend   Hominy Man;
   Minigeman   Raising crops
   Soholgol   He began.

26 Sakimawtenk   The next sachem was
   Alkosohit   The Subdivider;
   Sakimachik   These sachems
   Apendawi   Were helpful.

27 Sakimawtenk   The next sachem was
   Shiwapi   Shriveled Man;
   Sakimawtenk   The next sachem was
   Penkwonwi   Drought.

28 Attasokelan   There was no rain,
   Attaminin   No food to gather;
   Wapaniwaen   Eastward they went
   Italissipek   To where there was water.

29 Oligonunk   Beyond the pass,
   Sisilaking   In the herd country,
   Nallimetzin   They found food
   Kolakwaming   In the Great Plains.

30 Wtenk-penkwonwi   After Drought,
   Wekwochella   Exhaustion;
   Wtenknekama   After him was
   Chingalsuwi   The Hardened One.

31 Wtenknekama   After him was
   Kwitikwond   The Denouncer,
   Slangelendam   Rebellious and
   Attagatta   Unwilling.

32 Wundanuksin   In anger,
   Wapanisham   Leaving eastward,
   Allendyachick   Some went away
   Kimimikwi   In secret.

Harvest and Dispersal

Book IV: verses 25 through 32

The Lenape way of life changed, centering on the raising and gathering of plant foods, perhaps including corn (IV:25). The Great Plateau region abounds in edible roots, wild fruits, and grains. It lies at the northern boundary of the area in which corn can be cultivated. (Corn is known to have been grown in the Southwest as early as 3500 B.C.) In addition, the Great Plateau has rivers, especially the Columbia, through which pass great salmon migrations that can support large numbers of people.

Life was good and the Lenape increased in numbers, spreading out into their new territory. This growth led to subdivisions into smaller units, and the clan structure was reorganized to take the new divisions into account (IV:26). But then the rains stopped, and the growth of the tribe was cut short. A great drought gripped the land (IV:27). The rivers dried up. The green plants withered. The Lenape people were sadly reduced in numbers and in strength. The survivors resolved to move on, toward the dawn (IV:28), in search of a new home beyond the high wall of the Rocky Mountains. There, they found food and new hope in the hunting country of the High Plains (IV:29).

As the Lenape slowly regained their strength, they spread out along the primarily eastward-flowing watersheds, the Saskatchewan, leading northeast, and the Missouri-Yellowstone, tending southeast. But the earlier divisions, combined with the toll of the drought, had destroyed their national unity (IV:30).

Generations passed without anyone worthy of being called a sachem. Hardened One (IV:30) tried to enforce unity, but he was followed by the Denouncer (IV:31), who was stubborn and violent. The Denouncer angered a large portion of the Lenape, who resolved to go their own way, breaking away (IV:32) to continue on into the East.

Two Algonquian-speaking tribes in California, the Yuroks and the Wiyots, may have originated from the Lenape who remained behind in the Great Plateau after the main body crossed the Rockies to the East.[27] The many Lenape who continued eastward across the Great Plains may have followed the Saskatchewan watershed northward to become the ancestors of the Algonquian-speaking tribes of Canada, such as the Cree, the Algonkins, the Montagnais, and perhaps even the great Ojibwa nation.

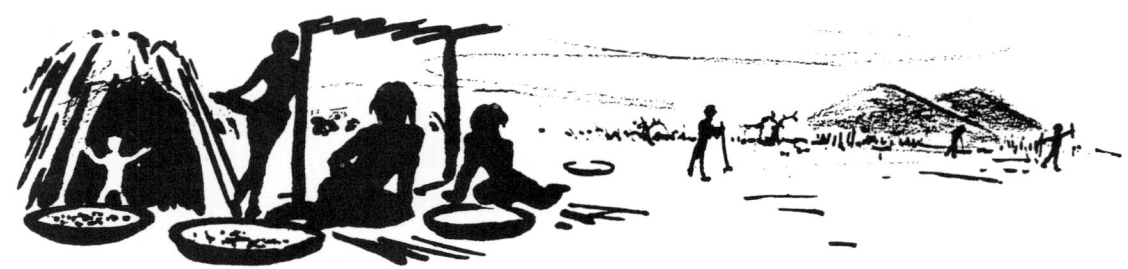

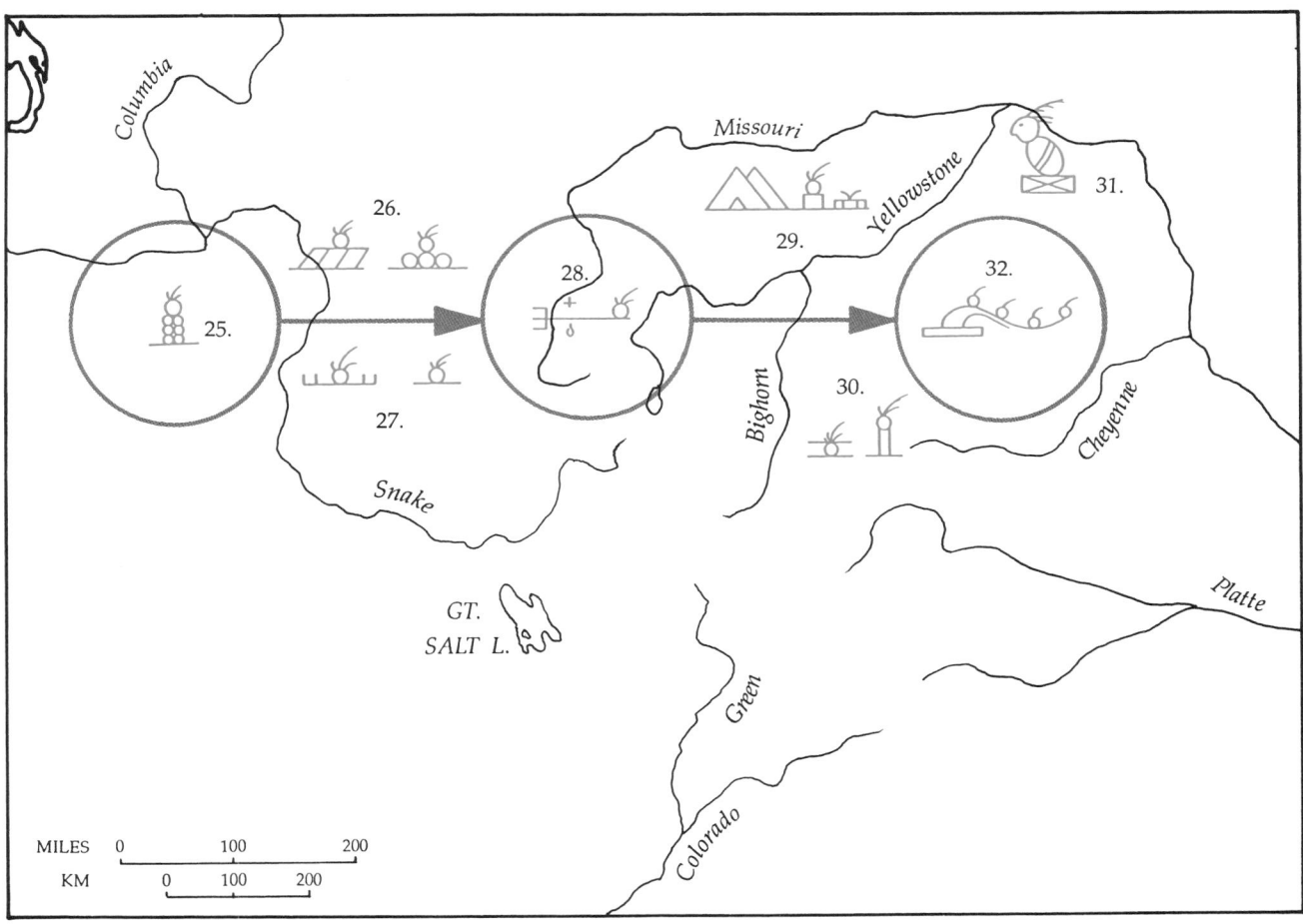

Figure 4.8. The map shows the migration route as revealed in verses 25 through 32 of Book IV. The numbers on the map and in the box below refer to the verses in which the symbols and location clues appear.

Location Clues

25. The Lenape are near the northern limit of where corn can be cultivated; the gathering of other plant foods may be implied here as well.

26. The sachem now is Subdivider. The process of subdivision of the tribe after its growth is echoed in other verses, including V:51–52, where once more there is a division into three parts.

27. Drought is characteristic of the Great Basin to the south, and periodic droughts have also affected the Great Plateau.

28. At this point, the scale of distance becomes three-quarters of the original distance (216 geographical miles) per step (see page 25). Note that the scale of the map here has been enlarged to make the steps appear the same size as before. The movement described here would take the Lenape across the Bitterroot Range of the Rockies, and across the Continental Divide.

29. Buffalo herds and other game animals are characteristic of the Great Plains.

30, 31. Note the absence of the mention of sachems, which indicates a lack of authority to hold the Lenape together.

32. From this location, the Missouri watershed flows away to the southeast. To the north, the Saskatchewan watershed leads in a different direction, to the northeast.

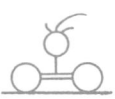

33 Gunehunga
   Wetatamowi
   Wakaholend
   Sakimalanop

   Remaining were
   The wise and prudent;
   The Beloved One
   They made sachem.

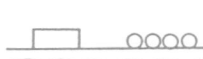

34 Wisawana
   Lappiwittank
   Michimini
   Madawasim

   By the Yellow River
   They settled again,
   Harvesting much
   From the wide meadows.

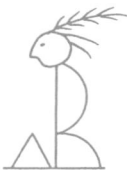

35 Weminitis
   Tamenend
   Sakimanep
   Nekohatami

   Everyone's friend,
   Tamanend
   Was the sachem,
   The first of that name.

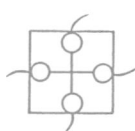

36 Eluwiwulit
   Matemenend
   Wemilinapi
   Nitispayat

   The best of all
   There was Tamanend;
   To all the Lenape
   He came as a friend.

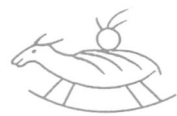

37 Wtenkwulitma
   Maskansisil
   Sakimanep
   W'tamaganat

   Thereafter it was good;
   Mighty Bison
   Was the sachem
   And the path-maker.

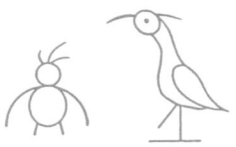

38 Machigokhos
   Sakimanep
   Wapkicholen
   Sakimanep

   The Great Owl
   Was the sachem;
   White Crane
   Was the sachem.

39 Wingenund
   Sakimanep
   Powatanep
   Gentikalanop

   The Willing One
   Was the sachem,
   Was the shaman,
   Making festivals.

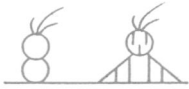

40 Lapawin
   Sakimanep
   Wallama
   Sakimanep

   Rich Again
   Was the sachem;
   Painted Red
   Was the sachem.

The Age of Peace

Book IV: verses 33 through 40

The Lenape who remained in the shelter of the mountains were wise and prudent. They elected a new sachem, the Beloved One (IV:33), who began to heal the wounds caused by the Denouncer (IV:31–32) and the departure of so many of their people. The new Lenape territory was centered on the fertile valley of the Yellow River (IV:34), which may be the Yellowstone. Around the source of this fertile watershed and hunting ground was a miraculous region from which sprang sacred power. To the east of the Yellowstone is the Black Hills, another sacred region.

After the Beloved One, Tamanend (IV:35), the first of three great chiefs to bear that name, became the Lenape leader. This name has sometimes been translated as "Wolf Man," but the more usual reading is "The Affable One." All of the admirable chiefs known as Tamanend were warmly remembered by the Delawares as paragons of ancient virtue: warmth, bravery, generosity, and openheartedness.[28] The second Tamanend is mentioned in V:32–33, the time period of this verse corresponds to a date around 1450. Tamanend the Third was the chief who later met William Penn for the Great Treaty in 1682.

Tamanend the First brought all the scattered Lenape people together in harmony (IV:36), uniting them into one nation. A happy age of prosperity and peace began, featuring great hunts and festivals. Mighty Bison (IV:37) was next; he was both a political leader and a spiritual leader or path-maker, with a special connection to the sacred buffalo.

The Willing One (IV:39) was the next leader. He acted as both sachem and shaman, presiding over great festivals where the people would gather together to give thanks for their blessings through prayer, singing, and dancing. The spirits of the Lenape rose and their influence spread (IV:40).

Lenape tribes such as the Blackfoot, the Cree, the Arapahoe, and the Cheyenne still inhabit the Plains and the foothills of the Rockies. Their ancient customs and legends recall what may have been the Lenape way of life at this time.[29] The high Plains were always inhabited by hunters, especially in the north. The bow and arrow was introduced into the area around 500 A.D., which corresponds roughly to this period.[30] In the days before horses came to the Plains, buffalo were killed by driving them into great pit-traps called *piskun* by the Blackfoot.[31] Every part of this sacred animal could be used for food, clothing, and shelter, and for everything from glue to water buckets, from weapons to toys.[32]

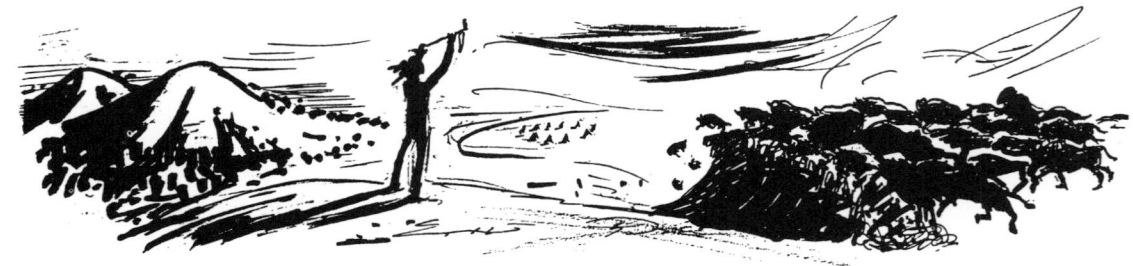

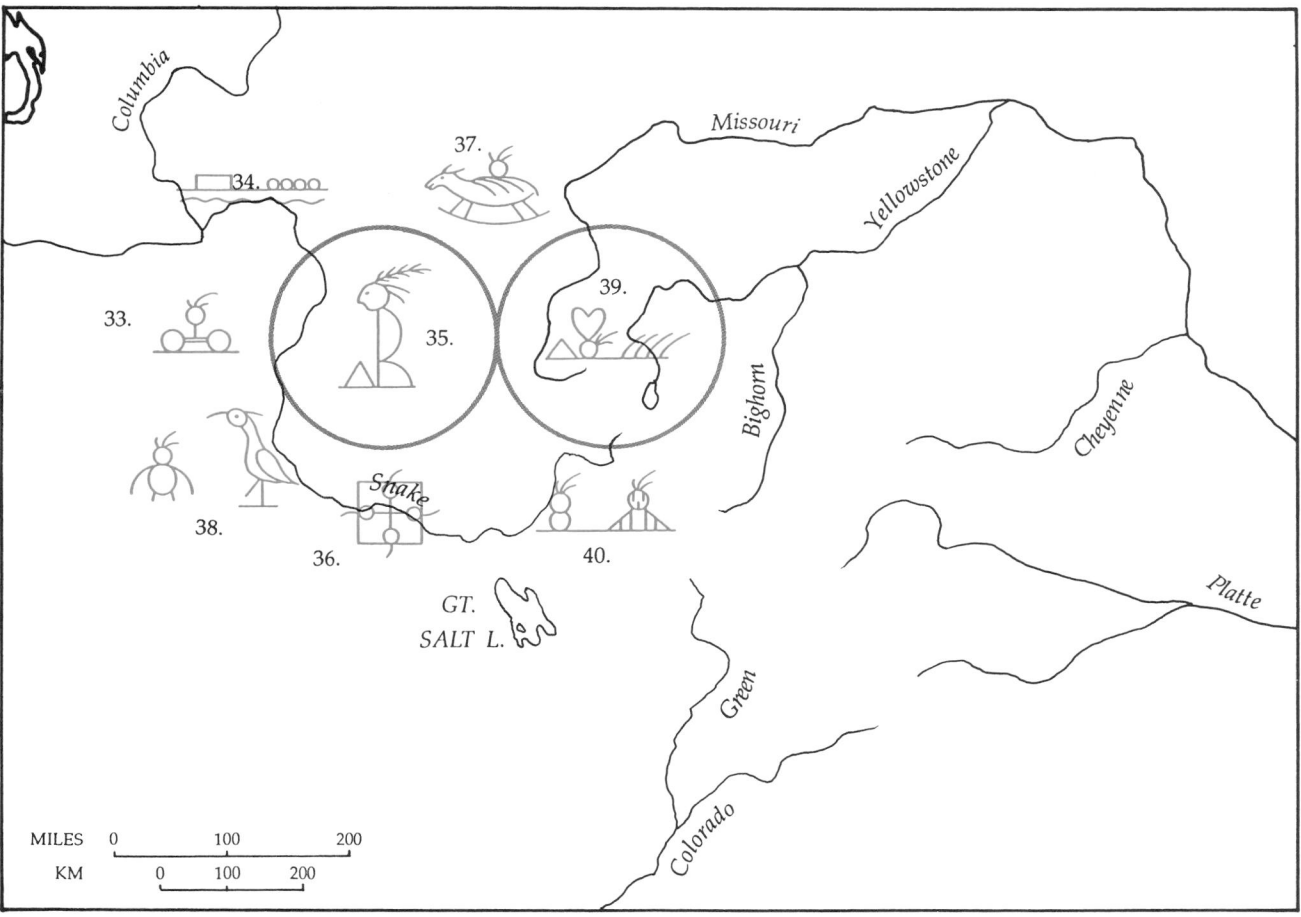

Figure 4.9. The map shows the migration route as revealed in verses 33 through 40 of Book IV. The numbers on the map and in the box below refer to the verses in which the symbols and location clues appear.

Location Clues

33. During this period, the Lenape were located among the foothills of the Rockies, near the Black Hills.

34. In this verse, the location might be the Yellowstone River. "Settled again" suggests a return of at least some of those who had left earlier (IV:32).

35, 36. Tamanend represents a unifying leader, a peacemaker capable of bringing the scattered Lenape groups together again.

37. Now Mighty Bison is sachem. Nomadic life on the aboriginal Great Plains depended heavily on following the buffalo herds.

38. Two sachem are mentioned in this verse: Great Owl and White Crane. The great grey owl is a large owl common in the northern forests; the location indicated on this map is the southern limit of its range. The whooping crane is a large white crane that was once common on the Great Plains, migrating north and south, like the buffalo.

39. Some movement is indicated in this verse, bringing the center of the Lenape population eastward to the intersection of the Missouri and the Cheyenne.

40. The names "Rich Again" and "Painted Red" both suggest success and prosperity.

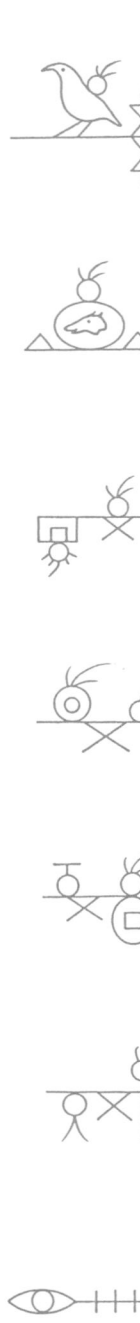
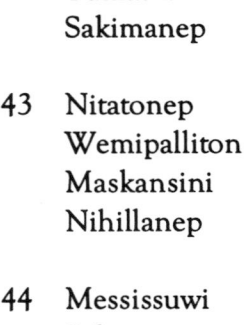

41 Waptipatit   White Chick
    Sakimanep   Was the sachem;
    Lappimahuk   Once more, bloodshed,
    Lowashawa   North and south.

42 Wewoattan   Wise and crafty
    Menalting   In council,
    Tumaskan   Mighty Wolf
    Sakimanep   Was the sachem.

43 Nitatonep   He could
    Wemipalliton   Fight every foe;
    Maskansini   The Strong Stone
    Nihillanep   He struck down.

44 Messissuwi   Whole-Hearted
    Sakimanep   Was the sachem
    Akowini   Fighting
    Pallitonep   The Snakes.

45 Chitanwulit   Strong is Good
    Sakimanep   Was the sachem
    Lowanuski   Fighting
    Pallitonep   The North Walkers.

46 Alokuwi   Poor One
    Sakimanep   Was the sachem
    Towakon   Fighting
    Pallitonep   Invaders.

47 Opekasit   East Looking
    Sakimanep   Was the sachem,
    Sakkelendam   Melacholy about
    Pallitonepit   The war there was.

48 Wapagishik   "To the Rising Sun
    Yuknohokluen   Now you must go," he said;
    Makelohok   Many were those
    Wapaneken   Who eastward went.

Widening War

Book IV: verses 41 through 48

The golden age of Tamanend finally ended in bloodshed, both in the north and in the south (IV:31). When warfare broke out during the time of White Chick, no enemy tribe is identified as the cause, as elsewhere in the Red Record; instead, the evidence points to this being a civil war. In contrast to White Chick, whose name is a symbol of weakness, the next leader who arises is Mighty Wolf, whose symbol (IV:42) shows him "between two fires." He is described as being crafty and able to fight everyone, so presumably a divided nation would be no disadvantage to him.

Mighty Wolf's slain enemy is identified as Strong Stone (IV:43). If Strong Stone were a rival Lenape leader, he might have been a false prophet; his symbol has a headdress of straight lines, like the headdress of the ancient Lenape shown in Book III, and there are five lines instead of the more common three, as on the holy man called the Prophet (V:13). If Strong Stone were a non-Lenape, it would be the only identification of a non-Lenape person by name in the Red Record. In this case, he might have been a leader of the Stonies, identified as an enemy tribe (V:16) that may be one of the Siouan-speaking tribes, such as the Assiniboines or the Lakota, which still inhabit the Great Plains.

Strong Wolf's success did not bring peace. Generation after generation of war followed, with the Lenape warriors fighting against invading tribes. These enemies may be related to the tribes that still can be found on the Great Plains: the Snakes

(IV:44) may represent Siouans or Shoshonean-speaking tribes, and the Invaders (IV:46) may represent either Siouans or Athabascan-speaking people.[33] The North Walkers (IV:45) have a symbol that matches the symbol for the Iroquoian-speaking Wyandots (IV:61, V:48) from the Great Lakes region; the Iroquoian-speaking people may have been located more to the west at this time.

Lenape victories became mixed with costly defeats. The future seemed to offer only more war and bloodshed as the Lenape faced an ever-increasing price for their territory beside the Rockies. But East Looking saw an escape, a vision of hope toward the dawn, where they were destined to find a better home. Inspired by this vision, the Lenape determined to leave, and they set off eastward on the long journey across the Great Plains. According to Delaware legend, it was on the Plains that they first encountered, and befriended, the people with whom their fate would be intertwined: the Iroquoians.[34]

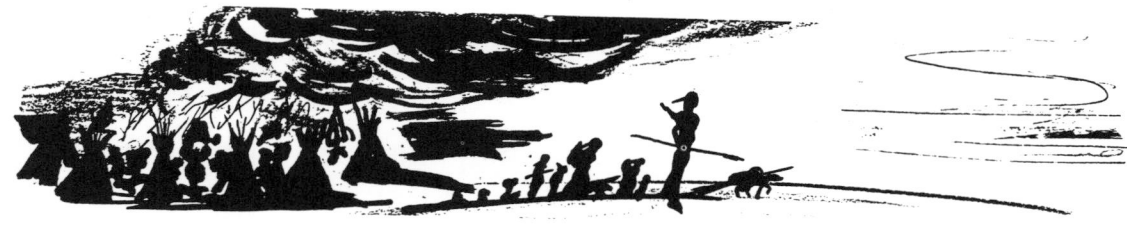

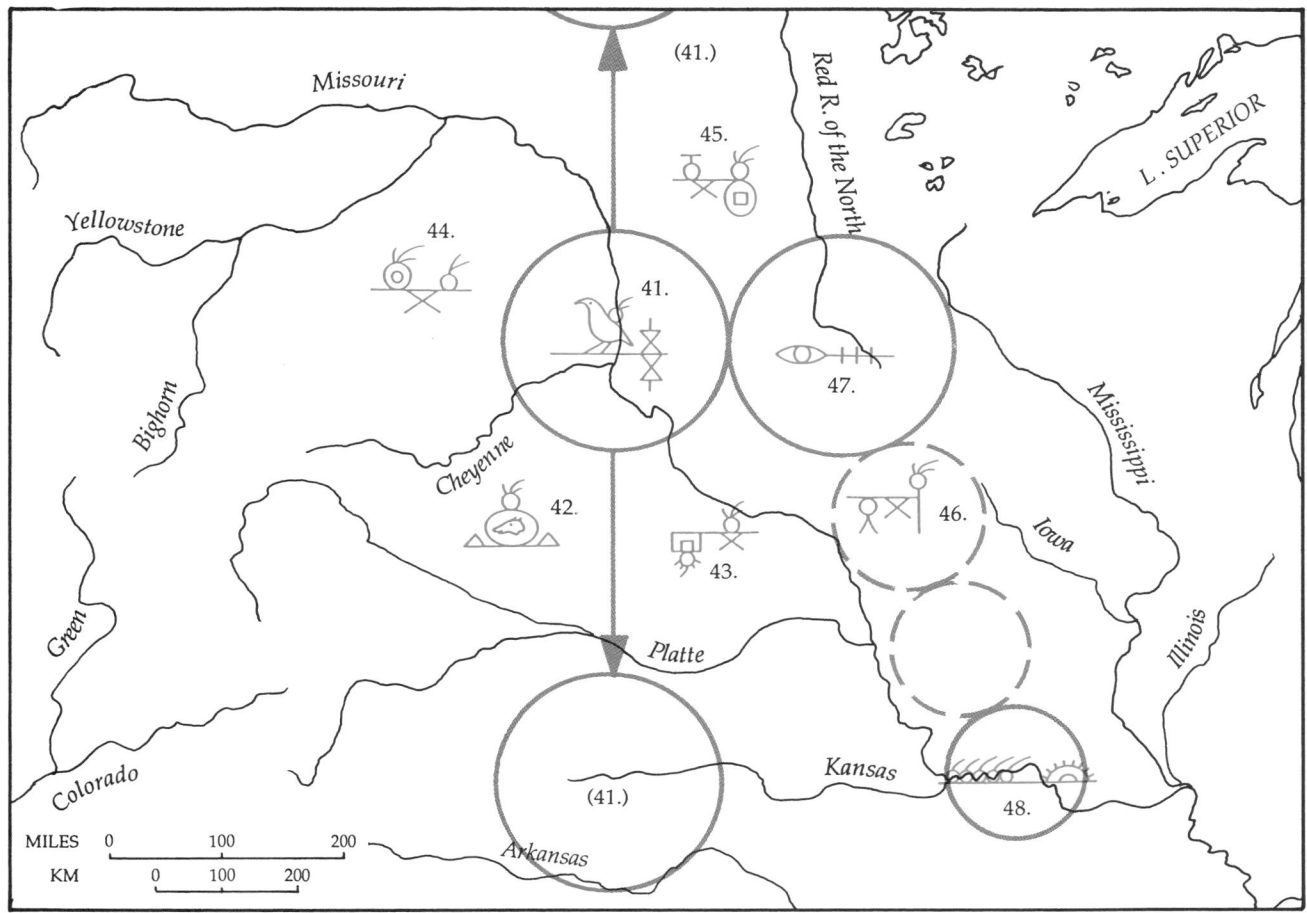

Figure 4.10. The map shows the migration route as revealed in verses **41** through **48** of Book IV. The numbers on the map and in the box below refer to the verses in which the symbols and location clues appear. Broken-line circles indicate that the movement has been inferred by the author rather than directly stated in the words and/or symbols.

Location Clues

41. The indications of north and south in this verse define a span of the Great Plains from Manitoba to Kansas. The greater prairie chicken, which resembles the symbol, once had a range almost identical to this area.

42. In this verse, Mighty Wolf is the sachem. The timber wolf, largest of the American wolves, was originally found as far south as this location.

43, 44. The Snakes might be from Siouan-speaking tribes (generalized location).

45. The symbol for the North Walkers is later used to describe the Wyandots, so they might have been an Iroquoian-speaking tribe coming west from the region of the Great Lakes.

46. The "Invaders" could either be Siouans or relative latecomers to the Great Plains such as the Athabascan-speaking tribes.

47. Their position astride the Great Plains left the Lenape vulnerable to raids from migrating tribes to the north and south.

48. The scale of distance changes from three-quarters to one-half of the original distance per step.

49	Tsehepieken	They separated
	Nemaissipi	At the Mississippi;
	Nolandowak	The lazy ones
	Gunehunga	Remained behind.
50	Yagawanend	The Lodge Man
	Sakimanep	Was the sachem;
	Tallegewi	The Talega
		[Moundbuilders]
	Wapawullaton	Possessed the East.
51	Chitanitis	Strong Ally
	Sakimanep	Was the sachem;
	Wapawaki	Land to the east
	Gotatamen	He asked for.
52	Wapallendi	Eastward some
	Pomisinep	Traveled;
	Talegawil	The Talega king
	Allendhilla	Massacred them.
53	Mayoksuwi	United, enraged,
	Wemilowi	All declared,
	Palliton	"To battle!
	Palliton	Destroy them!"
54	Talamatan	The Iroquois,
	Nitilowan	Their northern friends,
	Payatchik	Then arrived
	Wemiten	To join them.
55	Kinehepend	Sharp One
	Sakimanep	Was the sachem,
	Tamaganat	The path-maker
	Sipakgamen	Across the river.
56	Wulatonwi	They won
	Makelima	Many victories there,
	Pallihilla	Driving away
	Talegawik	The Talegas.

Collision With the Moundbuilders

Book IV: verses 49 through 56

As they neared the Mississippi, the Lenape people came upon agricultural lands where permanent settlements became possible. These settlements were characterized by earth lodges, which is reflected in the name and symbol of the next leader, Lodge Maker (IV:50).[35] Farther to the east were the powerful people called the Talegas. The origin of "Talegas" is still unclear. The word can perhaps be best translated as "foreigner" or "stranger." The Talegas were probably of the Muskogean language family, which lived throughout most of the Southeast.

Delaware traditions, as recorded by Heckewelder, describe this period in some detail, permitting a fuller understanding of events in the Red Record. According to Heckewelder, the Lenape arrived at the Mississippi and followed it downstream to where it meets the Missouri River. This is the location of Cahokia, the most likely site for the "Talega king" in IV:52. The great walled city of Cahokia, near where East St. Louis is today, was a commercial, political, and religious center of the last and most spectacular era of Moundbuilder culture—the Mississippian Temple Mound phase.[36] Cahokia has been described as "a cross between New York, Washington, D.C., and the Vatican."[37]

From the banks of the Mississippi, the Lenape sent a message to the Talegas, requesting permission to settle in their neighborhood as friends and allies. The Talega king denied this request, but promised to permit the Lenape to pass through his lands to find homes farther east. Peacefully, the Lenape began to cross the Mississippi. But when the Talega king saw how numerous the Lenape were, he became frightened, and ordered his warriors to attack. Talega war canoes swept across the river as armored Talega regiments massacred the Lenape who had already crossed. Enraged by this treachery, the Lenape vowed to "Conquer or die!" and joined with their Iroquois allies in an epic war of vengeance.[38] Led by Sharp One (IV:55), the Lenape forces stormed across the Mississippi, defeating the Talegas, and besieging and capturing many of the Talega towns.

Anthropologists agree that a last glimpse of the Talega way of life, known as the Mississippian Culture, was preserved by the Natchez of Mississippi. The Natchez had an absolute king, known as the Great Sun, who ruled over a society of rigid classes: the Lesser Suns, the Nobles, the Honored Men, and, at the bottom, the peasants and laborers known as the Stinkers. They built great earthworks and pyramids as bases for their temples. Their pursuit of status and power sometimes led them to commit human sacrifices. They were probably the most absolutist tribal society known north of Mexico.[39] Such a society of rigidity, privilege, and slavery would seem to be the temperamental opposite of Lenape society, which stressed individualism, freedom, and equality.

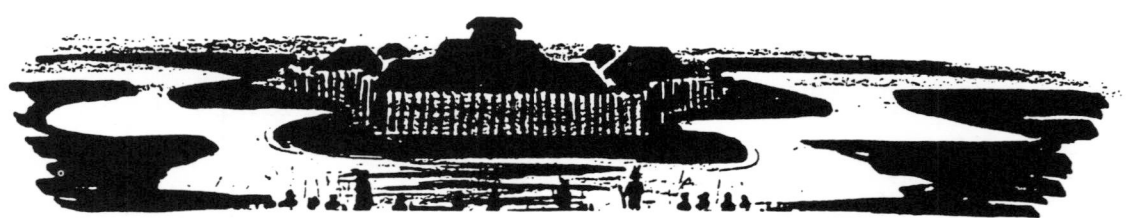

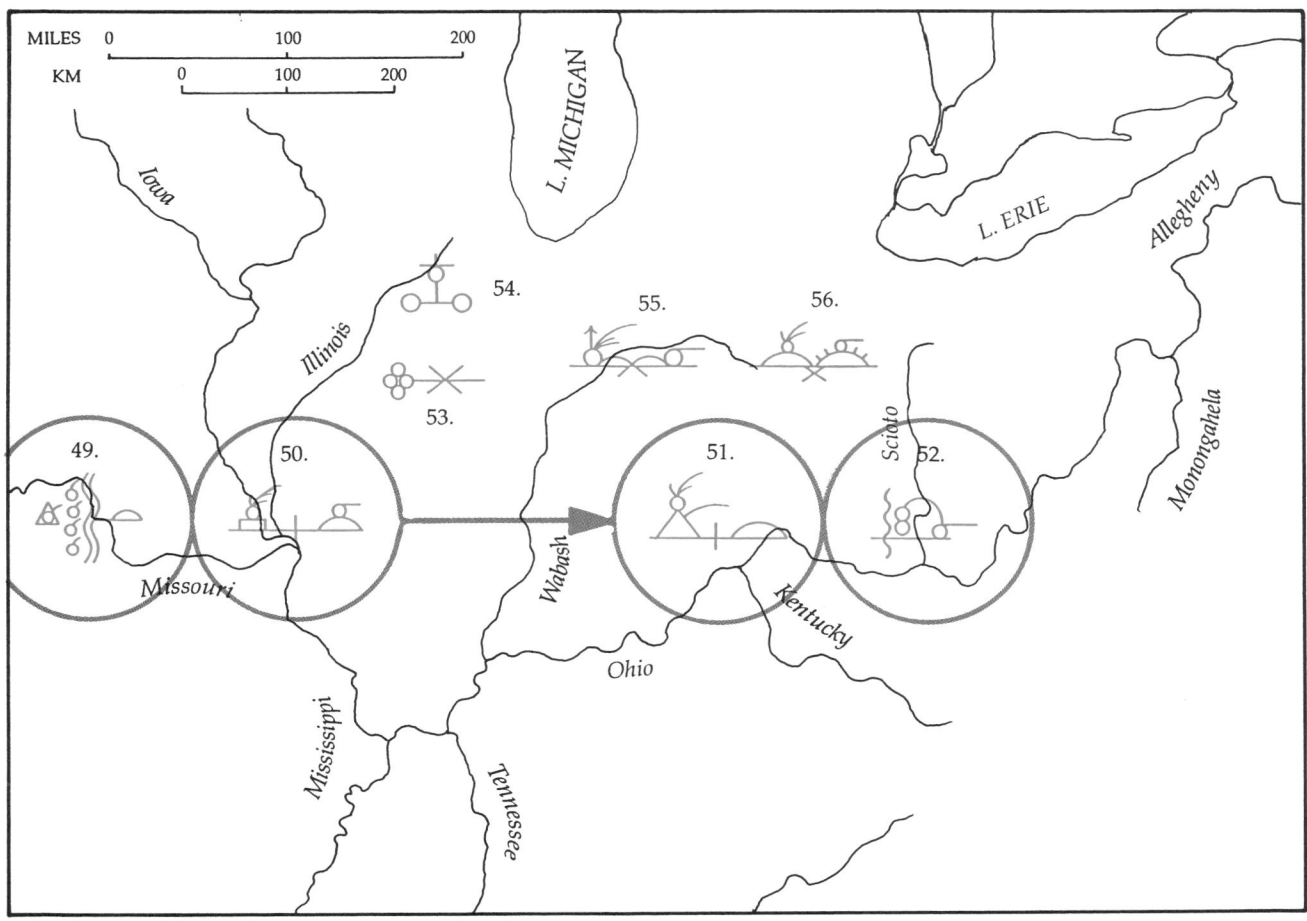

Figure 4.11. The map shows the migration route as revealed by verses **49** through **56** of Book IV. The numbers on the map and in the box below refer to the verses in which the symbols and location clues appear.

Location Clues

49. Differing lifestyles of western nomadic hunters and farmers of the lower Missouri are reflected.

50. Now, Lodge Maker is sachem. Earth lodges were characteristic of aboriginal farmers of the western prairie. The Moundbuilders represented an agrarian culture found throughout the Ohio valley and the middle and lower reaches of the Mississippi. The location at this point matches the location of the great Moundbuilder city of Cahokia.

51. The indicated movements would take the Lenape into the heart of the Moundbuilder culture.

52. However, the symbol, as well as Delaware legend, indicates that these events took place more to the west, after the Lenape attempted to cross the Mississippi.

53. Four symbols of the Lenape are shown united for war, the same number as shown on the banks of the Mississippi in IV:49.

54. Although "Talamatan" indicates the Wyandots from the central Great Lakes region, traditional Iroquoian allies of the Lenape, the symbol for the eastern Iroquois is used, so the translation is always given based on the symbol.

55, 56. The river mentioned here is most likely the Mississippi, but it could be the Illinois or even the Wabash, which would take the Lenape into the heart of the Moundbuilder culture in the east.

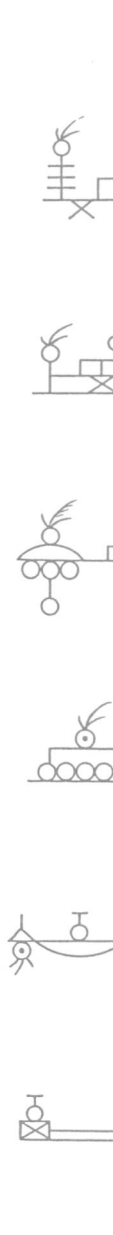

57 Pimokhasuwi   Stirring
     Sakimanep   Was the sachem;
     Wsamimaskan   Extremely strong were
     Talegawik   The Talegas.

58 Tenchekensit   Breaking Open
     Sakimanep   Was the sachem;
     Wemilat   Capturing all
     Makelinik   The great towns.

59 Paganchihilla   The Crusher
     Sakimanep   Was the sachem;
     Shawanewak   Southward fled
     Wemitalega   All the Talegas.

60 Hattanwulaton   Having Possession
     Sakimanep   Was the sachem;
     Wingelendam   Jubilant were
     Wemilennowak   All of the people.

61 Shawanipekis   South of the Great Lakes
     Gunehungind   We lit our fires;
     Lowanipekis   North of the Lakes were
     Talamatanitis   Our Wyandot friends.

62 Attalechinitis   But they were not
                       true friends
     Gishelendam   And conspired;
     Gunitakan   Long in the Woods
     Sakimanep   Was the sachem.

63 Linniwulamen   Truthful Man
     Sakimanep   Was the sachem
     Pallitonep   Who fought against
     Talamatan   The Iroquois.

64 Shakagapewi   Righteous
     Sakimanep   Was the sachem;
     Nungiwi   Trembling were
     Talamatan   The Iroquois.

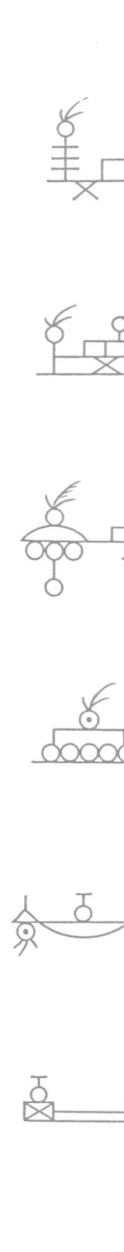
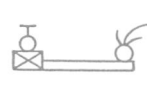
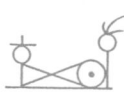
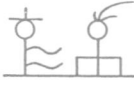

Victors and False Friends

Book IV: verses 57 through 64

After a long and difficult struggle, Talega resistance was crushed (V:57–59). The Red Record shows that four sachems came and went before the final victory (V:55–59). The war between the Lenape-Iroquois allies and the Talega must have been fierce, with the final sieges of the Talega Wars among the largest battles ever fought in ancient America. Formidable earthworks from this period can be found throughout the Ohio Valley. One such stronghold, Fort Ancient, had pallisaded walls 13 feet high and 5 miles long, and could hold up to 10,000 people.[40]

For both the Lenape and the Iroquois, the usual method for dealing with captives would have been to make them run the gauntlet to prove their mettle; then, if they could find a sponsor, the captives would be adopted into the tribe.[41] In this way, the tribes grew by assimilation.

The defeated remnants of the Talega fled southward, never to return (V:59). The Natchez were among the descendants of the Talega who fled down the Mississippi River. Natchez legends told of a time when the people had lived far up the Mississippi to the north and east.

The victorious Lenape took possession of a new homeland (V:60). After the Lenape-Iroquois victory, the land was divided, with the Iroquois in the north, around the Great Lakes, and the Lenape in the south, along the Ohio Valley (V:61). But the Lenape's erstwhile allies, the Iroquois, were "not true friends," and tried treacherous attacks upon the Lenape under Long In The Woods (IV:62); they were stopped and punished by

Truthful Man (V:62). The quarrel between the Lenape and the Iroquois may have arisen because of conflicts over hunting rights, unsolved murders, or, as the Red Record suggests, a secret plot. In a Delaware legend, it is told how the Iroquois once started a war between the Lenape and the Cherokees by murdering a Cherokee child and leaving a Lenape war club as evidence.[42] Once the cycle of revenge and counter-revenge was begun, it was often very difficult to stop. Whatever happened, the Lenape remained estranged from the Eastern Iroquois, later to become the Six Nations, whom they called the Mengwe (the Pricks) but remained friendly with the Wyandots of Canada, whom they called the Talamatans.

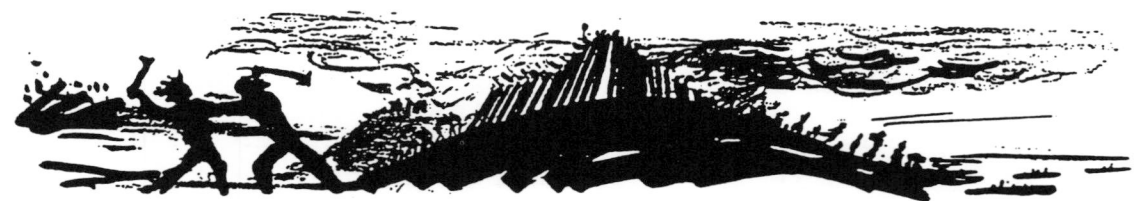

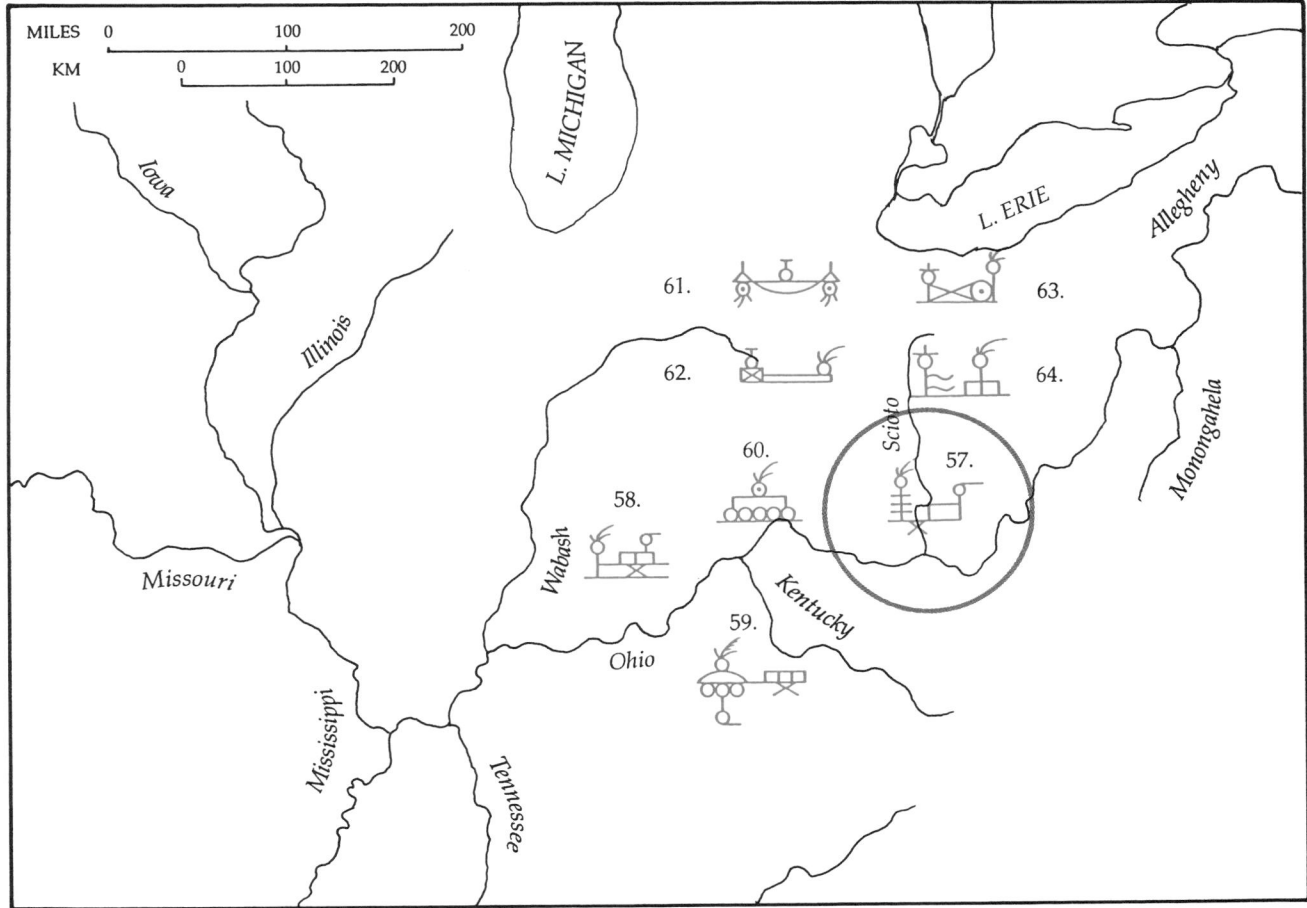

Figure 4.12. The map shows the migration route as revealed by verses **57** through **64** of Book IV. The numbers on the map and in the box below refer to the verses in which the symbols and location clues appear.

Location Clues

57. The Lenape are now located in the heart of the Moundbuilder culture of the upper Ohio valley, near such famous Moundbuilder sites as Fort Ancient. No additional migrations are indicated in this chapter.

58. The "great towns" are symbolized by squares.

59. Legend has the Talega fleeing down the Mississippi. Note that in the symbol, the Talega have abandoned their towns and are in the south.

60. This symbol shows a Lenape holy man atop an establishment supported by a large number of people.

61. The division of territories was probably made according to watersheds. The Wyandots were traditional allies of the Lenape.

62. The mention of forests reflects the fact that the Lenape were now in the Eastern Woodlands.

63. The symbol shows a sacred presence or person shielding the Lenape chief in his fight against the eastern Iroquois.

64. The Lenape tribes came to dominate the western Great Lakes, while the Iroquoians maintained control of the eastern half.

Book V

Symbols	Original Words	Translation
	1 Wemilangundo Wulamotalli Talegaking	All was peaceful, Long ago, there In the Talega country.
	2 Tamaganend Sakimanep Wapalaneng	The Path Maker Was the sachem Beside the Shining Stream.
	3 Wapashuwi Sakimanep Kelilgeman	White Lynx Was the sachem, Growing great crops.
	4 Wulitshinik Sakimanep Makelopannik	Fine Forests Was the sachem; The people were many.
	5 Lekhihitin Sakimanep Wallamolumin	The Author Was the sachem, Writing the Red Record.
	6 Kolachuisen Sakimanep Makeliming	Pretty Bluebird Was the sachem; There were great harvests.
	7 Pematalli Sakimanep Makelinik	Always There Was the sachem; The towns were many.
	8 Pepomahemen Sakimanep Makelaning	Navigator Was the sachem Along many streams.
	9 Tankawon Sakimanep Makeleyachik	Little Cloud Was the sachem; Many were those who left.
	10 Nentegowi Shawanowi Shawanaking	The Nanticokes [and] The Shawnee Went to the south land.

The Family Multiplies

Book V: verses 1 through 10

A new age began, an age of peace. The Lenape explored their new homeland, a land of deep forests laced by many rivers such as the Wabash, the White or Shining River, in what is now Indiana (V:2). The Lenape called their new homeland the Talega Country (V:1), in memory of the people who had once lived there.

In the soft soil of the river bottoms, in fields cleared by the men and tended by the women, the Lenape grew flourishing crops (V:3) of the life-giving combination of corn, beans, and squash. Nourished by the bounty of this new land, the people multiplied (V:4), and the Lenape family grew.

It was a time of rest and reflection, a time to recall their proud past. So the Author (V:5), drawing upon records dating back as far as History Man (IV:23), added the most recent events to the chronicle called the Wallam Olum, the Red Record.

In this time of abundant harvests (V:6), new Lenape towns and villages appeared throughout the Ohio valley (V:7). Well-worn footpaths connecting them were frequented by visitors and traders. Traders' canoes followed the many streams (V:8) leading into the Ohio (the Talega River) and the Mississippi (the "Gathered Waters"). Trade networks extended for hundreds of miles, and precious objects might travel for thousands. Shoppers in the markets of the Midwest could choose among items from the East Coast to the Rockies, from Canada to the Gulf of Mexico.[43]

But then the harvests failed. It was the time of Little Cloud (V:9), a time of drought and hunger. As the crops shriveled, the answer for a large number of hungry Lenape families lay to the south, beyond the Ohio in the hunting preserve of what is now Kentucky. They broke away and became the tribes known as the Nanticokes and the Shawnee (V:10). The Nanticokes, who had a reputation for using sorcery, would find their way through the Cumberland Gap into Virginia, and eventually settle in the tidelands of Maryland. The vigorous and courageous Shawnee, the Southerners, would travel deep into the South along the valleys of the Appalachians.

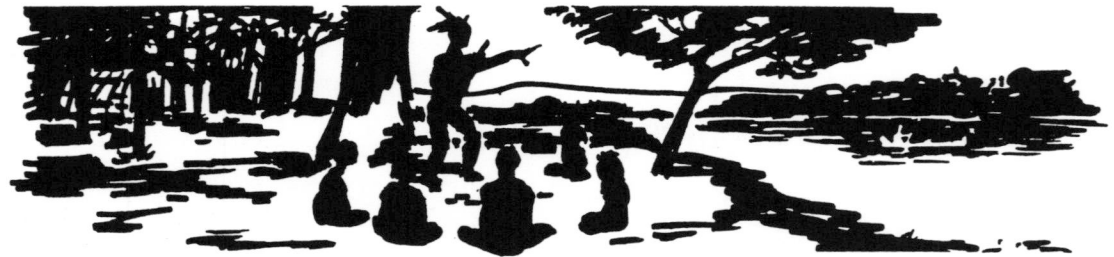

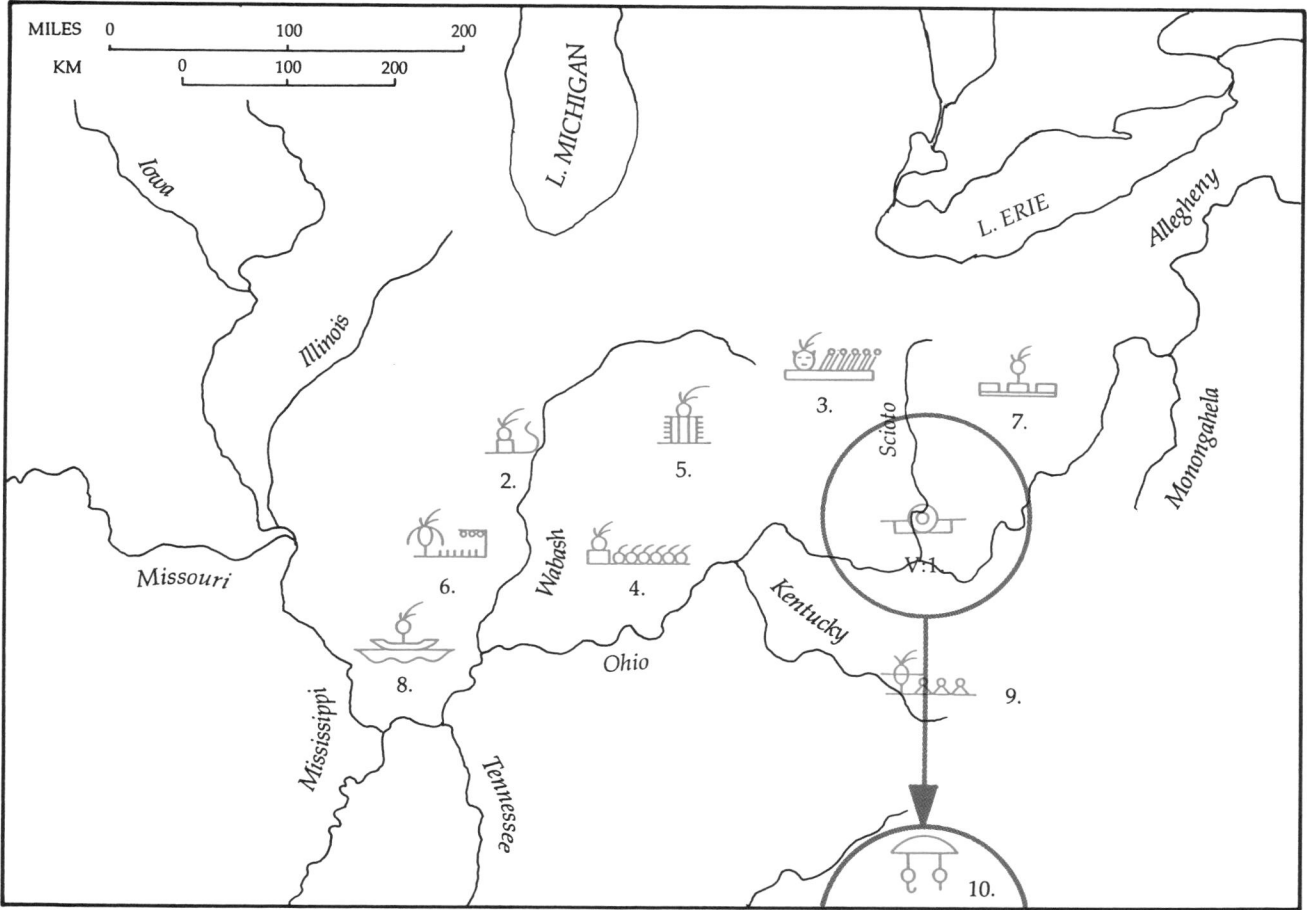

Figure 4.13. The map shows the migration route as revealed by verses 1 through 10 of Book V. The numbers on the map and in the box below refer to the verses in which the symbols and location clues appear.

Location Clues

1. The Lenape remain centered in the upper Ohio Valley, referred to here as "the Talega Country."

2. "Shining Stream" suggests either the Wabash or the White River in Indiana, which can both be translated similarly.

3. In this verse, the sachem is White Lynx. The Canadian lynx is light-colored, but is seldom seen south of the Great Lakes; a darker, smaller cousin, the bobcat, can be found farther south, but is still rare in the Midwest, except in the lower Ohio valley and along the middle reaches of the Mississippi.

4. Again, the magnificent forests characteristic of the Eastern Woodlands are mentioned.

5. This is the location where Dr. Ward received the Red Record in 1820.

6. Here, during the reign of Pretty Bluebird, there are "great harvests." Blue songbirds common to this area include the Eastern bluebird, the indigo bunting, and the barn swallow, which nests in buildings such as those where harvests are stored.

7. The Midwest was more populous than the regions west of the Mississippi, and life centered on settled villages.

8. The Ohio-Mississippi-Missouri watershed connected a vast area, opening it to travel and trade.

9,10. The Shawnee had territories below the Ohio, in Kentucky and farther south.

11	Kichitamak Sakimanep Wapahoning	Great Beaver Was the sachem At the White Salt Lick.
12	Onowutok Awolagan Wunkenahep	The Prophet, Seer of heaven, Went westward.
13	Wunpakitonis Wunshawoshonis Wunkiwikwotank	West, to those left behind; West, to those in the south; West, visiting all there.
14	Pawanami Sakimanep Taleganah	Rich Turtle Was the sachem Along the Ohio.
15	Lokwelend Sakimanep Makpalliton	Traveler Was the sachem; There was bad war.
16	Lappitowako Lappisinako Lappilowako	Again, the invader Snakes; Again, the stony Snakes; Again, the northern Snakes.
17	Mokolmokom Sakimanep Mokolakolin	Canoe Master Was the sachem Fighting the foe in boats.
18	Winelowich Sakimanep Lowushkiakiang	Hunter in Snow Was the sachem Through the northern wastes.
19	Linkwekinuk Sakimanep Talegachukang	The Beholder Was the sachem Through the Alleghenies.
20	Wapalawikwan Sakimanep Waptalegawing	Eastern Home Was the sachem East of the Ohio.

Storm Clouds Gather

Book V: verses 11 through 20

By regrouping in their hunting territories, the Lenape tried to recover from the effects of the drought (V:11). In hunting territories, salt licks were especially valuable as the place where game animals would gather.

A great holy man, the Prophet, "seer of heaven" (V:12), went back to the west to visit the Lenape who had been "left behind" (V:13) nineteen generations before (IV:48–49), when the Lenape went eastward to their fateful encounter with the Talegas. (In the Rafinesque Manuscript and here, the first symbol for the Prophet has seven lines in the headdress, and five lines in the second symbol.)

Fearlessly, the Prophet crossed the Great Plains to visit the Lenape's distant relatives near the Rocky Mountains, from the north into the south. Near the southern relatives were the great pueblo towns of the Anasazi, the Old Ones, ancestors of the modern pueblo tribes. The Anasazi people had a flourishing culture at this time, with advanced strains of corn. Perhaps the Prophet traded for some of this drought-resistant corn, for prosperity returned to the Talega Country under Rich Turtle (V:14), a name that refers to the Lenape's survival of the great Flood in II:9–16.

But other dangers were on their way. Migrating tribes began to attack travelers and enter into Lenape territories (V:15). These tribes were among those the Lenape had fought long ago: the Shoshonean, Siouan, and possibly Athabascan tribes, their old enemies from the Rockies and the Great Plains (V:16).

Using the mobility afforded by rivers and streams, sleek Lenape birchbark canoes carrried Lenape warriors in every direction (V:17), including north to the northern lakes of Michigan and Wisconsin. The expansion of the Lenape northward into the Great Lakes region, probably accompanied by a shift of the Iroquoian tribes away to the east, led eventually to the establishment in the area of many Lenape tribes, such as the Menominee, Potowatomi, Ottawa, Sauk, Fox, and perhaps the Ojibwa.

Far to the north, in the snowy wastelands beyond the northern forests, was a new foe (V:18). The Lenape relatives north of the Great Lakes, such as the Cree, Montagnais, and Algonkins of Canada, called them the Eskimos, "Eaters of Raw Meat."

To the east of the Alleghenies, the "Talega Mountains," explorers found a new opportunity, perhaps because a migration of the native population at this time left this inviting region relatively uninhabited. According to legend, a sachem of this era left his realm to his two sons. When one son made war upon the other, the latter departed with his people in search of a new home.[44] These two sons could be the sachems mentioned in verses 19 and 20—note that the symbol for the Beholder (V:19) resembles that in IV:47, where war also triggered a migration.

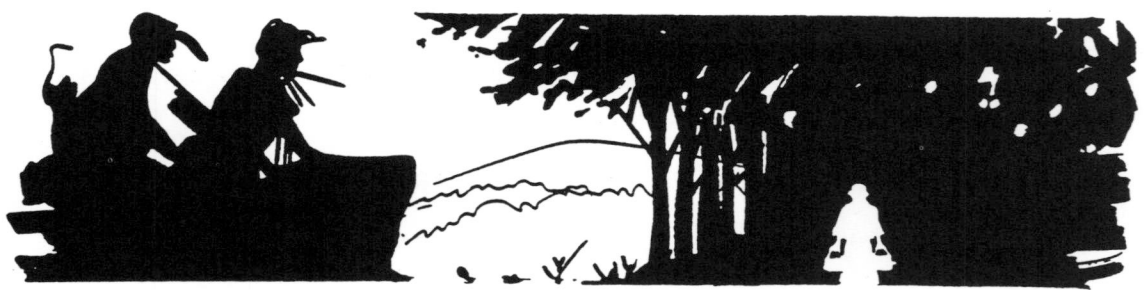

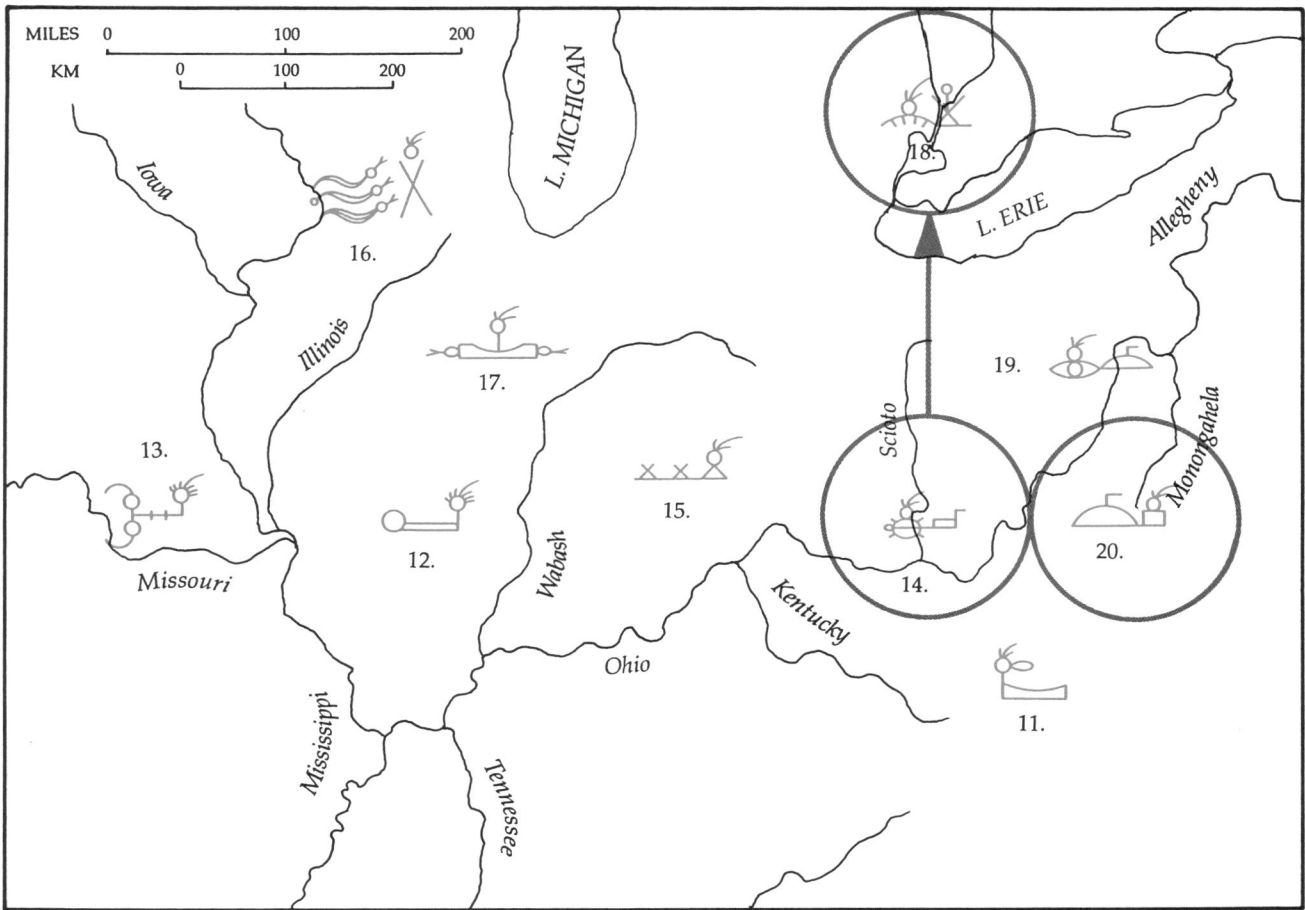

Figure 4.14. The map shows the migration route as revealed in verses 11 through 20 of Book V. The numbers on the map and in the box below refer to the verses in which the symbols and location clues appear.

Location Clues

11. Great Beaver is now sachem. Beavers are found throughout subarctic North America. The "White Salt Lick" could be the Great Salt Lick in Kentucky, or some other salt lick in the Midwest.

12, 13. Since the travels of the Prophet are identified as a "visit," the main body of the Lenape is left in place in the Talega Country. Those that the Prophet visited were the Lenape "left behind" on the Great Plains, north and south.

14. The Lenape are in the Talega Country; they called the Ohio the Talega River.

15. The symbol implies that the fighting was in the west.

16 . The names of the Lenape's enemies are the same as those from the Great Plains, and implies an invasion from that region.

17. Whether the fighting here refers to a campaign in the Minnesota "Land of Lakes" or elsewhere is uncertain. The symbol refers to an overall region rather than to a specific place.

18. Although the described movement only goes as far as Lake Huron, the verse may refer to events much farther north in Canada.

19. Here, the sachem rules over the Alleghenies, which are located in West Virginia and western Pennsylvania.

20. In this verse, the symbol shows a location east of the Alleghenies.

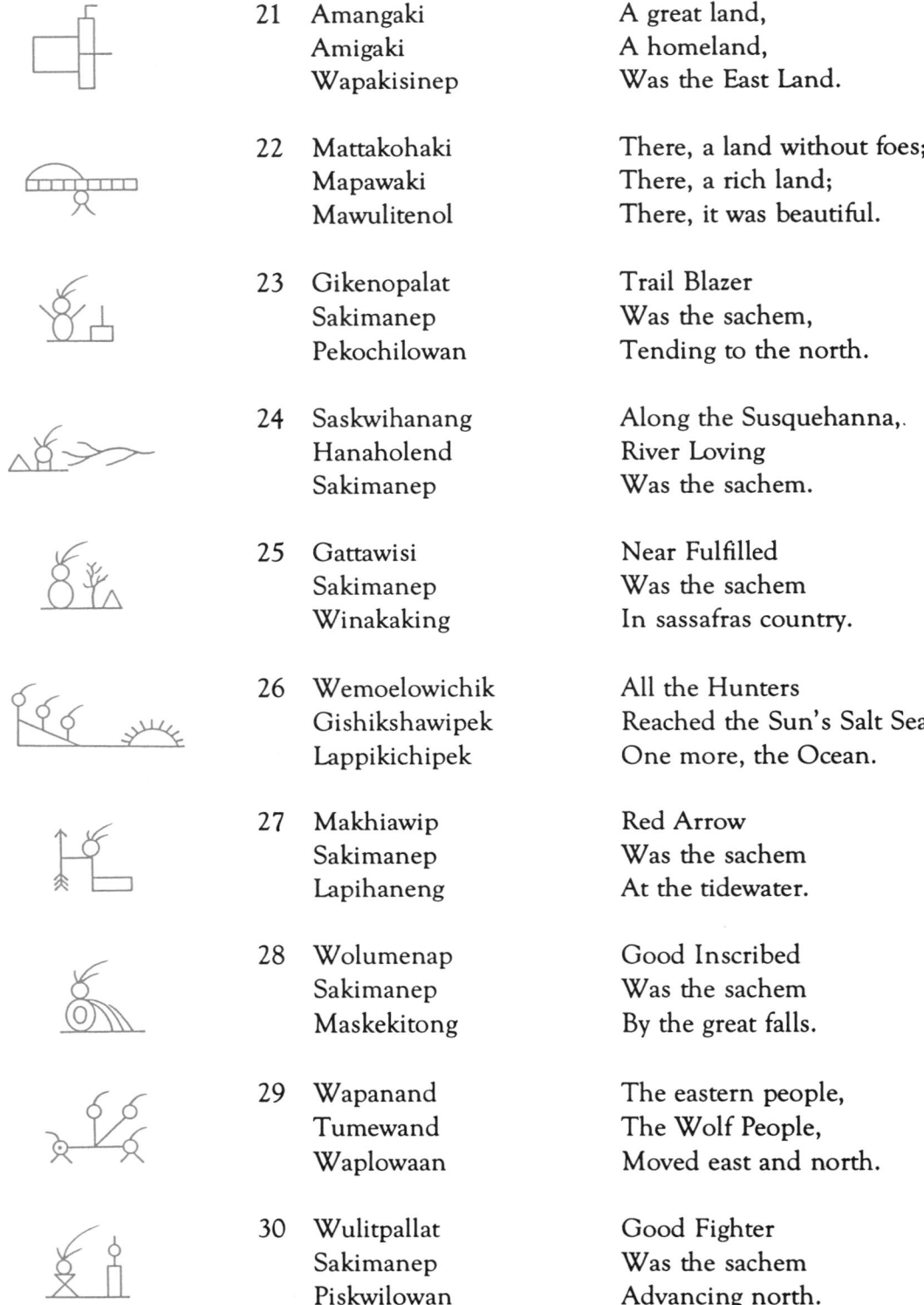

21 Amangaki
Amigaki
Wapakisinep

A great land,
A homeland,
Was the East Land.

22 Mattakohaki
Mapawaki
Mawulitenol

There, a land without foes;
There, a rich land;
There, it was beautiful.

23 Gikenopalat
Sakimanep
Pekochilowan

Trail Blazer
Was the sachem,
Tending to the north.

24 Saskwihanang
Hanaholend
Sakimanep

Along the Susquehanna,.
River Loving
Was the sachem.

25 Gattawisi
Sakimanep
Winakaking

Near Fulfilled
Was the sachem
In sassafras country.

26 Wemoelowichik
Gishikshawipek
Lappikichipek

All the Hunters
Reached the Sun's Salt Sea;
One more, the Ocean.

27 Makhiawip
Sakimanep
Lapihaneng

Red Arrow
Was the sachem
At the tidewater.

28 Wolumenap
Sakimanep
Maskekitong

Good Inscribed
Was the sachem
By the great falls.

29 Wapanand
Tumewand
Waplowaan

The eastern people,
The Wolf People,
Moved east and north.

30 Wulitpallat
Sakimanep
Piskwilowan

Good Fighter
Was the sachem
Advancing north.

To the End of the Earth

Book V: verses 21 through 30

Free, open, and spacious, the East beckoned the Lenape people (V:21). The East had peace and plenty, in a land without enemies (V:22). Delaware legends say that twice as many moved into the East as stayed behind in the Talega Country, and that this migration to the East took place over a period of forty years.

The Lenape worked their way northeastward through the dense forests, up the long valleys of the Alleghenies (V:23). They explored the branching watershed of the Susquehanna (V:24), and came at last into the beautiful green country (V:25) along the Delaware River (called the Lenape River), which lead down to the Great Eastern Sea. They stood at last on that sacred shore where the Earth each day received the first light of the dawn (V:26). They had reached the easternmost edge of the world, and found there the homeland of their dreams.

Here was the happy ending to one of the longest recorded migrations in human history—over 9,000 miles from Asia to the East Coast of America. To commemorate this event, a special calendar belt of black wampum was started, with a new bead added every year. When the beads were counted later, this belt showed that the Lenni Lenape had arrived at the East Coast in 1396.[45] This eastward journey to a happy home may have been the result of an age-old dream or prophecy.

Before the Lenape moved across the Bering Strait, the east had been the land of their dreams. At this point in the Red Record, it says they are at the ocean "once more" (V:26); the symbol shows the sun rising from the water. The last ocean they had actually seen would have been the Pacific; the last time they had seen the sun rise above the ocean would have been on the Asian shore of the Bering Strait when the dawn revealed a miraculous bridge of ice leading to the New World. After the crossing, the Lenape are always pictured in the Red Record with a curved line above their heads, pointing to the east, the direction in which they faced when they prayed. (The Lenape word for east, *wapa,* means white and light and is similar to *pawa,* which means rich and powerful, in the sense of having strong dreams; this is the derivation of the word *powwow.*[46]) For the Lenape, the east was a force that pulled them forward; so long as they followed the rising sun, they would find what they were looking for.

Having arrived at the Atlantic Ocean, the Lenape now began a trek that would take them first north and then east again. From the heartland along the Delaware, the Lenape spread out to the northeast (V:29) and fought their way up the Hudson River Valley (V:30). Mohican legends say that when the Mohicans, a Lenape tribe, first saw the ebb and flow in the estuary of New York Harbor, they were reminded of the tides in a place like the Bering Strait.[47] This part of the migration opened the way for the Lenape settlers of the New England area, who would become such tribes as the Massachusetts, the Nipmuc, the Narraganset, the Pequot, the Wampanoag, the Montauk, and many others.

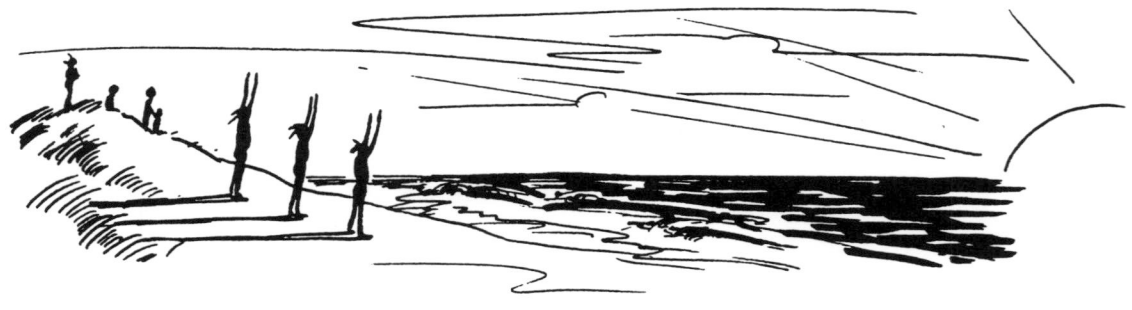

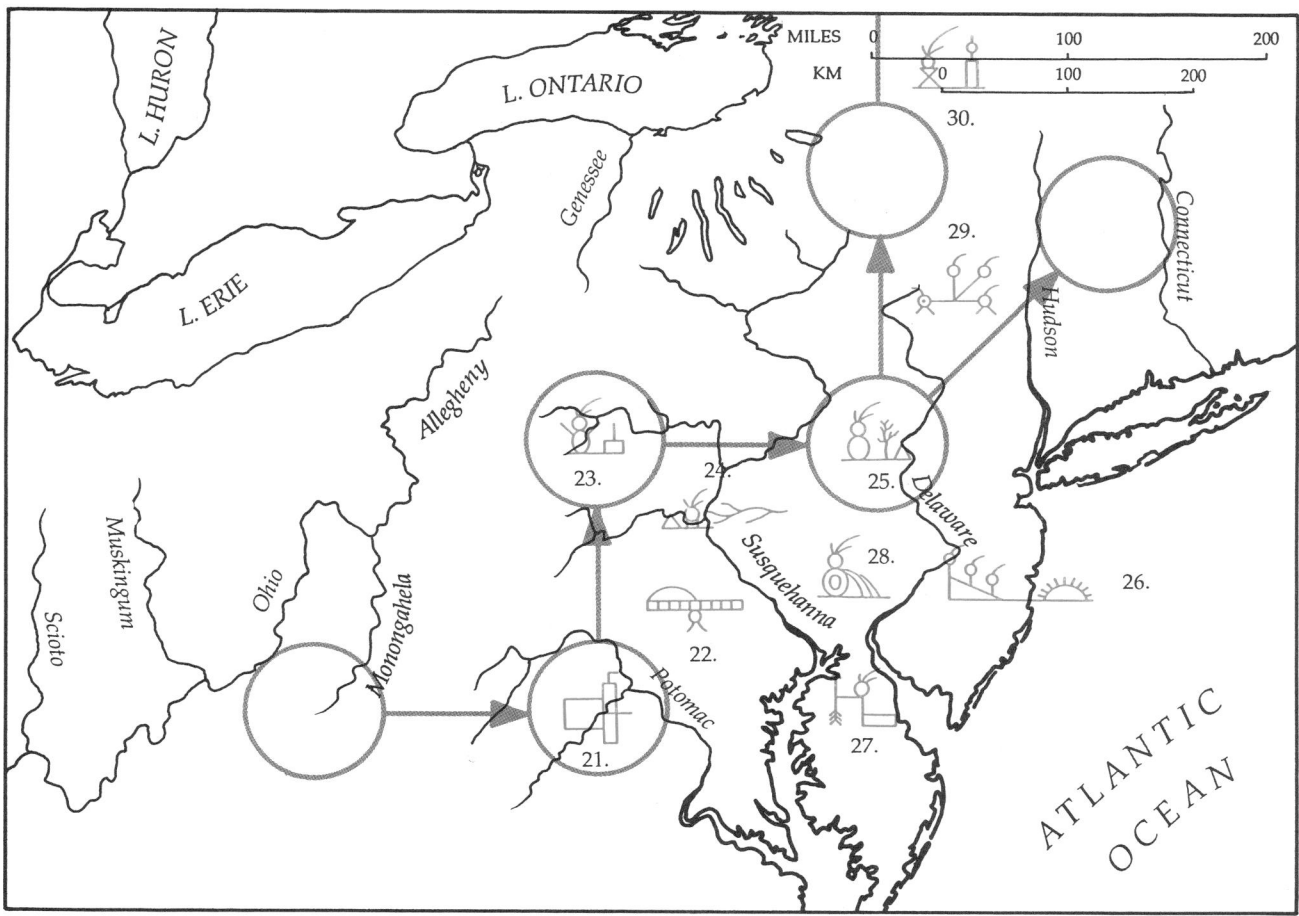

Figure 4.15. The map shows the migration route as revealed in verses 21 through 30 of Book V. The numbers on the map and in the box below refer to the verses in which the symbols and location clues appear.

Location Clues

21. Here the scale changes once again, from one half of the original distance per step to one third per step (see page 25).

22. The "land without foes" could reflect an absence of people, or the presence of relatives who were already living there.

23. The valleys of the Alleghenies run in a northeast direction. If only one northward step is charted, then the endpoint of the Lenape migration becomes exactly the same as the historical heartland of the Lenni Lenape.

24. The Susquehanna, the watershed for central Pennsylvania, is clearly identified.

25. Sassafras Country was the Lenape name for eastern Pennsylvania.

26. The Lenape reach the sea, somewhere along the shore of present-day New Jersey or Delaware.

27. The "tidewater" might be the point where the tides could be felt on the Delaware River.

28. The "great falls" could be farther upstream on the Delaware, at the transition between the mountains and the coastal plain.

29. The indicated movement leads along the eastern boundary of the territory of the Five Nations Iroquois and into New England.

30. This verse represents a movement up through Lake Champlain to Canada.

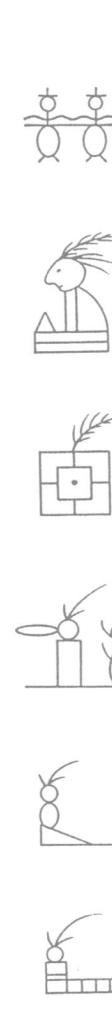

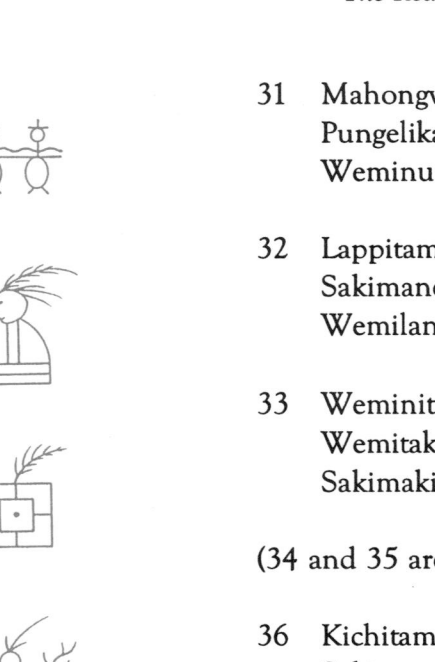

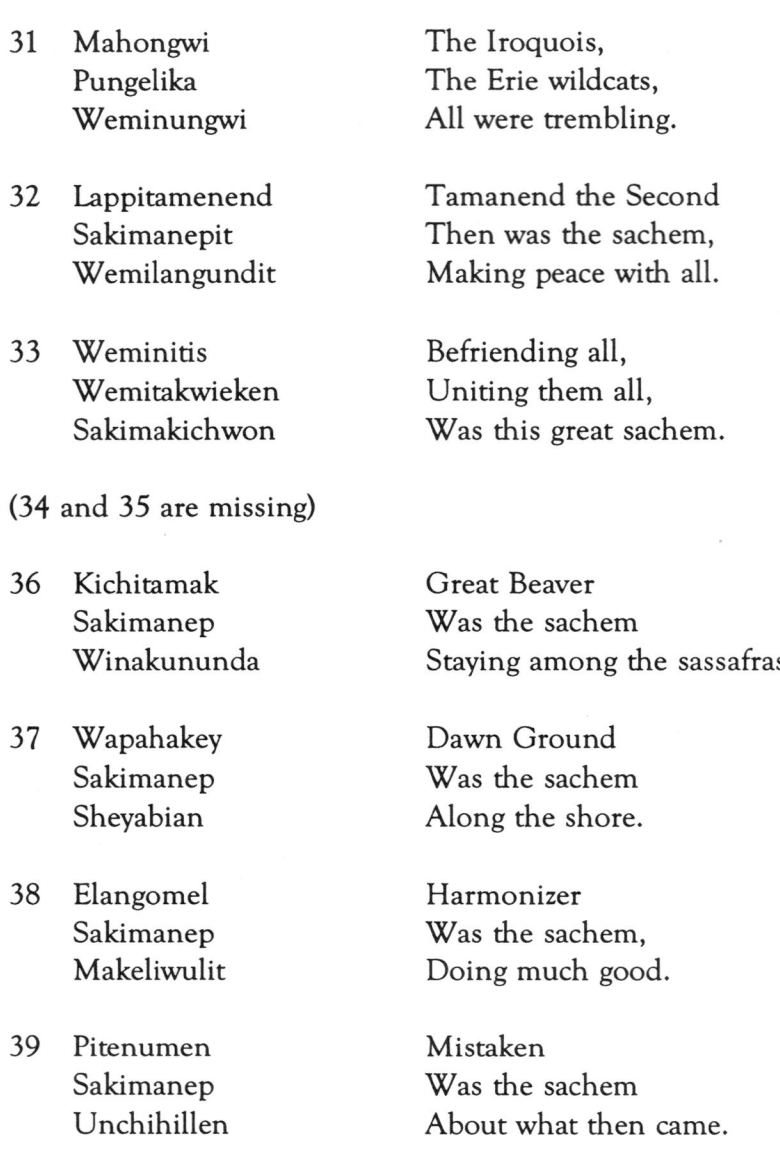

31	Mahongwi	The Iroquois,
	Pungelika	The Erie wildcats,
	Weminungwi	All were trembling.
32	Lappitamenend	Tamanend the Second
	Sakimanepit	Then was the sachem,
	Wemilangundit	Making peace with all.
33	Weminitis	Befriending all,
	Wemitakwieken	Uniting them all,
	Sakimakichwon	Was this great sachem.

(34 and 35 are missing)

36	Kichitamak	Great Beaver
	Sakimanep	Was the sachem
	Winakununda	Staying among the sassafras.
37	Wapahakey	Dawn Ground
	Sakimanep	Was the sachem
	Sheyabian	Along the shore.
38	Elangomel	Harmonizer
	Sakimanep	Was the sachem,
	Makeliwulit	Doing much good.
39	Pitenumen	Mistaken
	Sakimanep	Was the sachem
	Unchihillen	About what then came.
40	Wonwihil	For at this time,
	Wapekunchi	From the Dawn Sea,
	Wapsipayat	The Whites appeared.

In the Land of Light

Book V: verses 31 through 40

With the Lenape settlement of New England, the Iroquoian-speaking tribes were completely surrounded by the Lenape tribes. The symbol for the Iroquois in V:31, which—according to the count of generations—corresponds to a period around 1438, is the first reference to the Iroquois since the end of Book IV. The symbol uses for the first time the name *Mahongwi* (Mengwe), the Lenni Lenape name for the Six Nations Iroquois. At this time weak and divided, the Iroquois and their Erie relatives had good reason to fear the Lenape. Their response may have been the formation of the League of the Iroquois by Deganawidah and Hiawatha. This action would later have far-reaching consequences.

Once the Iroquois Five Nations, later to become Six, united, they would gradually grow in strength until, with the aid of the Dutch and the English, they would crush the other Iroquoian and Lenape tribes around them and dominate even the Delawares. The League form of government was admired by the Founding Fathers and served as a model for the federal government later set up in the United States Constitution. Though the date for the formation of the League is often set at 1579—possibly indicated in the symbol for V:48, which shows a unification involving the Iroquoian Wyandots—other authorities place the date at 1390 or even earlier.[48]

For the Lenni Lenape, the period described in these verses was for the Lenape a time of glory, the summit of their history. The great Tamanend the Second became sachem (V:32); he was the friend of all, and brought all the Lenape tribes together in peace (V:33). He may have had his capital along the Delaware River near Shackamaxon, "The Place Where Chiefs Are Made," close to present-day Philadelphia.

In the deep green forests, full of game, and in the wide bright shorelands along the great Eastern Sea, the Lenni Lenape lived happily (V:36); the sacred Pipe of Peace brought harmony to them all. Wampum beads, laboriously shaped from shells, were a spiritual as well as commercial medium of exchange, and would have meant considerable power for the shoreline tribes (V:37). The other medium of exchange was tobacco. The smoke of the pipe (V:38) wafted the feelings of the heart out to blend with those of the other smokers, and up to the watching spirits of the universe.

In such a time of harmony and spiritual fulfillment, it was a natural mistake for the Lenni Lenape to conclude that the unearthly strangers who floated in from out of the Eastern Sea in 1524 (V:39–40)[49] were visitors from the Spirit World, headed by the Great Spirit himself! (The native account of this momentous first encounter is retold on pages 140–144.)

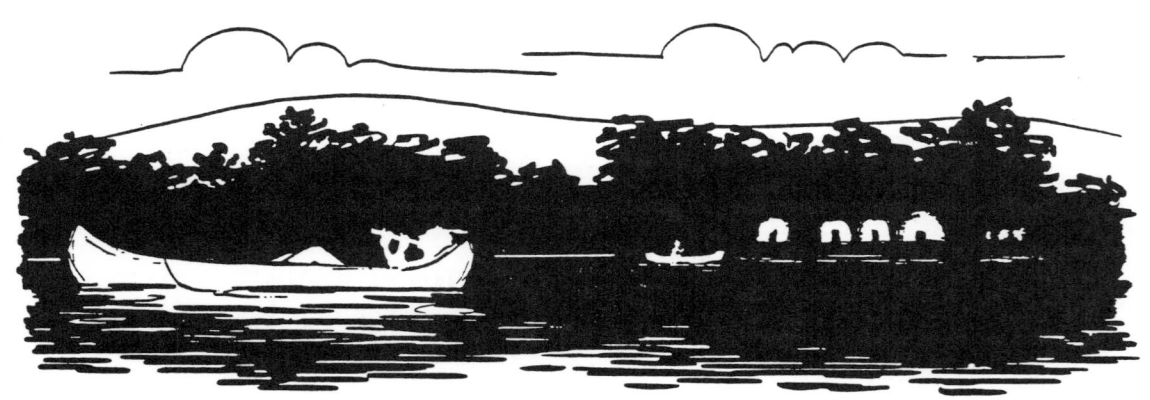

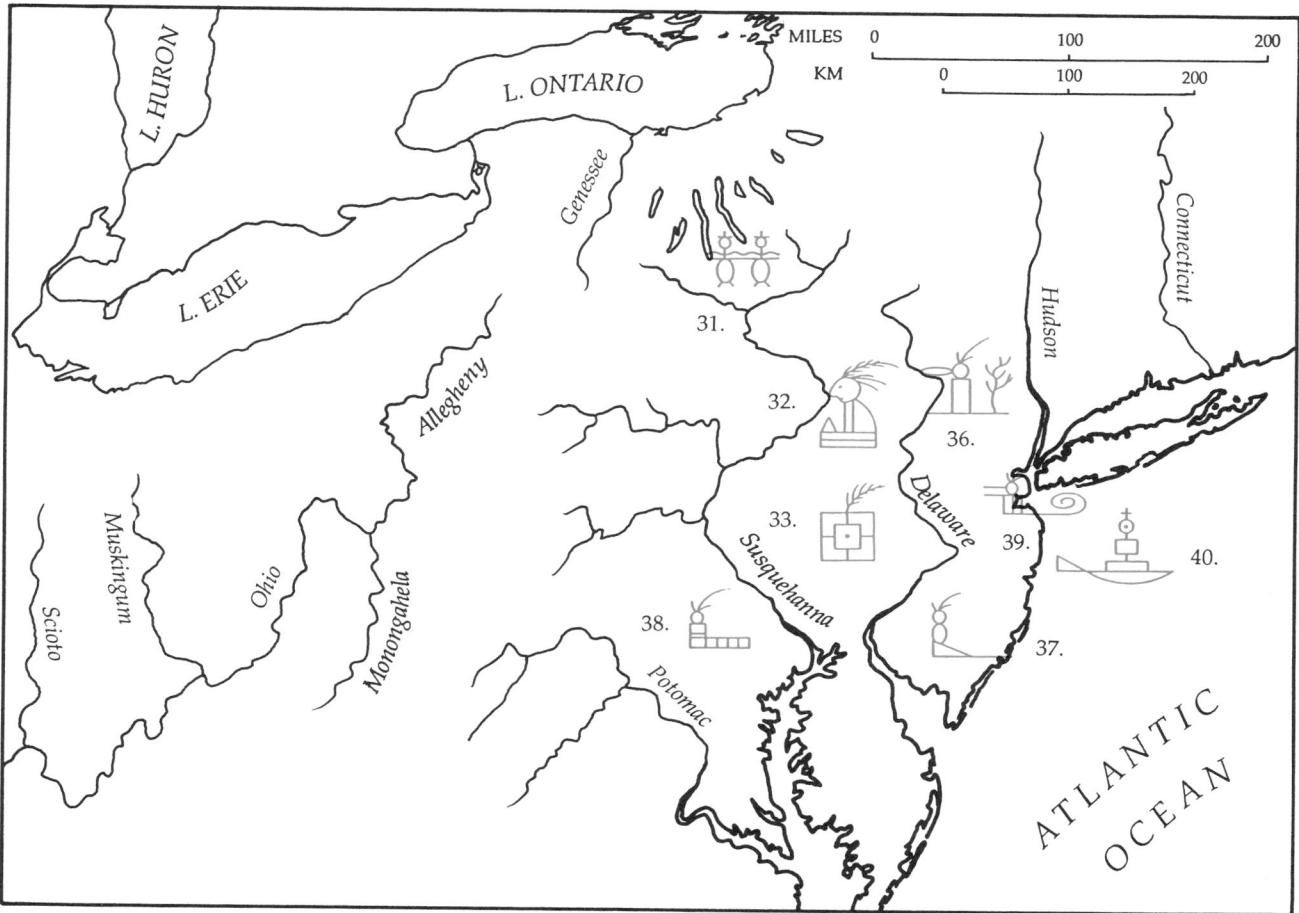

Figure 4.16. The map shows the migration route as revealed in verses **31** through **40** of Book V. The numbers on the map and in the box below refer to the verses in which the symbols and location clues appear.

Location Clues

31. Here the words clearly indicate the Five Nations Iroquois, whether or not they had achieved their union by this time. The Iroquoian-speaking Eries were a warlike tribe to the southeast, along the lake that bears their name.

32. At this point, the Lenape migration has ended (note the triple ground line in the symbol), so further indications of movement are deleted from the maps. The base location for the Lenni Lenape from here on is along the Delaware River.

33. The capital of the great Tamanend the Second is located here, near present-day Philadelphia.

36. Two verses seem to be missing; at least one of them seems to have described another division of the tribe (see III:12, IV:33, IV:49).

37. Here, along the eastern shore of the United States, fishing and harvesting of shellfish made another way of life possible. The manufacture of wampum beads brought wealth and prestige.

38. The symbol suggests a pipe, as well as a forest land (see V:22).

39. The two lines pointing to the left (westward) in the sachem's symbol echo the lines pointing eastward in the symbol for the whites in V:60.

40. The most probable location for the arrival of the whites is New York Harbor, where Verrazano appeared in 1524.

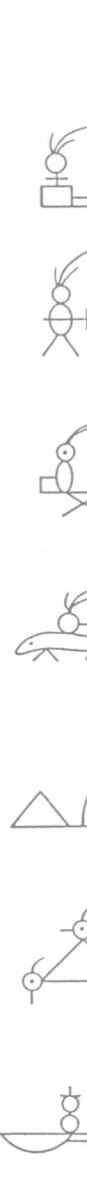

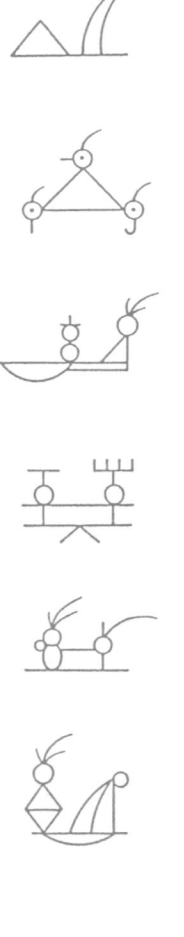

41 Makelomush
Sakimanep
Wulatenamen

Much Honored
Was the sachem,
And was happy.

42 Wulakeningus
Sakimanep
Shawanipalat

Well Praised
Was the sachem
Advancing into the South.

43 Otaliwako
Akowetako
Askipalliton

For over there were snakes;
Strongholds of the enemy
That must be destroyed.

44 Wapagamoshki
Sakimanep
Lamanitis

White Otter
Was the sachem,
Friend of the Wyandots.

45 Wapashum
Sakimanep
Talegawunkik

White Horn
Was the sachem
West to the Ohio.

46 Mahiliniki
Mashowoniki
Makonowiki

There, were the Illinois;
There, were the Shawnee;
There, were the Conoy.

47 Nitispayat
Sakimanep
Kipemapekan

Friend coming
Was the sachem
To the Great Lakes.

48 Wemiamik
Weminitik
Kiwikhotan

All their children,
All their friends,
They visited.

49 Pakimitzin
Sakimanep
Tawanitip

Cranberry Eating
Was the sachem;
The Ottawas were friends.

50 Lowaponskan
Sakimanep
Ganshowenik

North Walker
Was the sachem
At the Noisy Place
[Niagara].

Travels Among Friends

Book V: verses 41 through 50

The Lenape were powerful and honored (V:41). Their power opened the way for widespread travel among all of their many friends and relatives throughout the Eastern Woodlands. Well Praised (V:42) won fame in his battles against the Lenape enemies in the southern mountains, where the Siouan-speaking Tutelos and the mighty Iroquoian-speaking Cherokees could be found (V:43). These victories helped protect the Shawnee and the Lenape tribes of Virginia, and kept the Alleghenies and the Cumberland Gap open for access to the Lenape who lived farther west.

White Otter (V:44) went as ambassador northward, to open trade and travel to their Iroquoian friends, the Wyandots. In the Talega Country, the great sachem White Horn (V:45) assembled many of the most powerful Lenape tribes—the Illinois of the west, the Shawnee of the south, and the Conoy of the tidelands—in a great council (V:46). Lenape traders and ambassadors were welcomed throughout the Great Lakes (V:47–48), even in the country of the Ottawas (V:47). Tribal allies everywhere in the north were on the move, and at the neutral Great Falls of Niagara, the Lenape sachem North Walker (V:50) presided.

This age of movement may have been a response to changes caused by the growing presence of European explorers and colonists. Although explorers would not visit the Lenni Lenape territory again until 1610, the effects of the Europeans could already be felt. The exotic diseases they introduced—measles, venereal diseases, smallpox, etc.—roared like wildfire through native populations, which had no immunity to them. Estimates of the number of Native Americans killed by these diseases range from three to thirty million people.[50] Whole tribes were wiped out. Other tribes or European colonists moved into the depopulated areas.

But at the same time, European traders brought objects of tremendous usefulness, such as metal tools, which made life much easier for the native people. Tribal traders could make great profits exchanging these items with other tribes further inland. European weapons were also a great advantage in war.

The European presence also led to a rearrangement of the tribes. Movements of native people to and away from the Europeans in Florida, Maine, Quebec, Georgia, and Virginia caused many conflicts and adjustments among the tribes, conflicts in which the Lenni Lenape could act as mediators. A major conference center arose by Niagara Falls, which was a recognized neutral zone. It was also the site of intertribal trade and sports festivals.

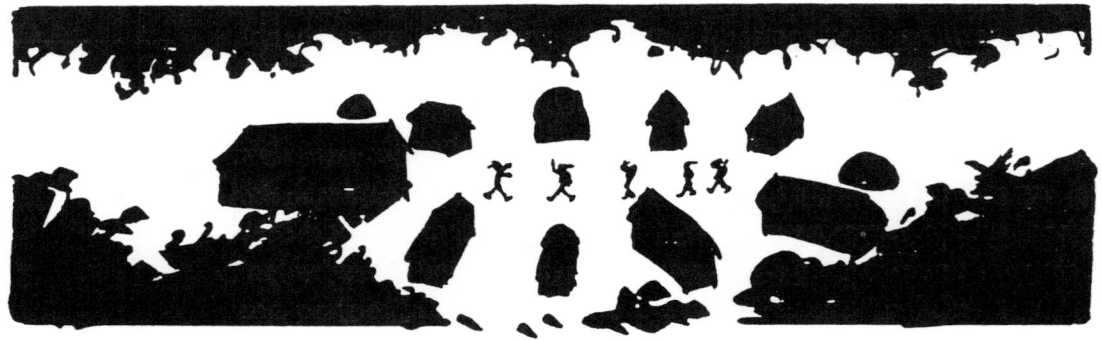

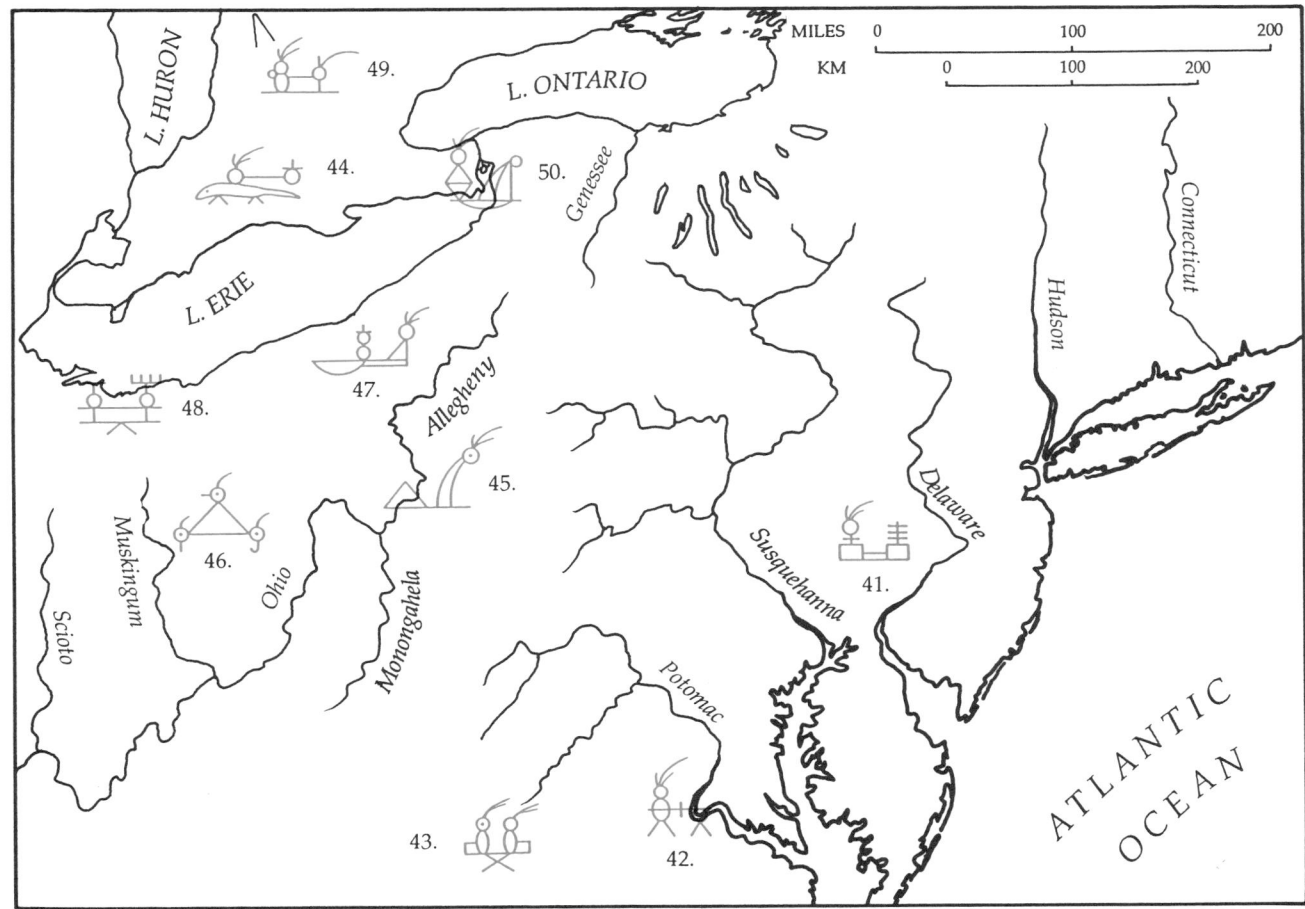

Figure 4.17. The map shows the location of the Lenape as revealed in verses 41 through 50 of Book V. The numbers on the map and in the box below refer to the verses in which the symbols and location clues appear.

Location Clues

41. The Lenape sachem displays the symbol for success, as in III:3 and IV:57.

42. This is the last described movement into a previously unmentioned area. It probably represents a campaign against foes in what is now Virginia.

43. The "Snakes" may be Siouan tribes that were found in the mountains of Virginia.

44. In this verse, White Otter is the sachem. The symbol shows the otter, a playful and intelligent denizen of rivers, and the Wyandots, who were based between Lake Huron and Lake Ontario. A white otter would be so unusual that it would be regarded as sacred, but around the Great Lakes, the weasel commonly appears in a white winter-phase, when it is known as an ermine.

45, 46. The Illinois, Shawnee, and Conoy tribes mentioned here represent the Lenape tribes of the west, the south, and the southeast. The Conoy were a Lenape tribe along the Potomac.

47. In order to open a direct route to the Great Lakes, the Lenni Lenape would have had to pass through the territory of the Eries.

48, 49. The Ottawas mentioned here originally occupied a territory near the junction of the lakes Huron, Superior, and Michigan. The symbol refers to an overall region rather than to a specific place.

50. In this verse, the location appears to be around Niagara Falls.

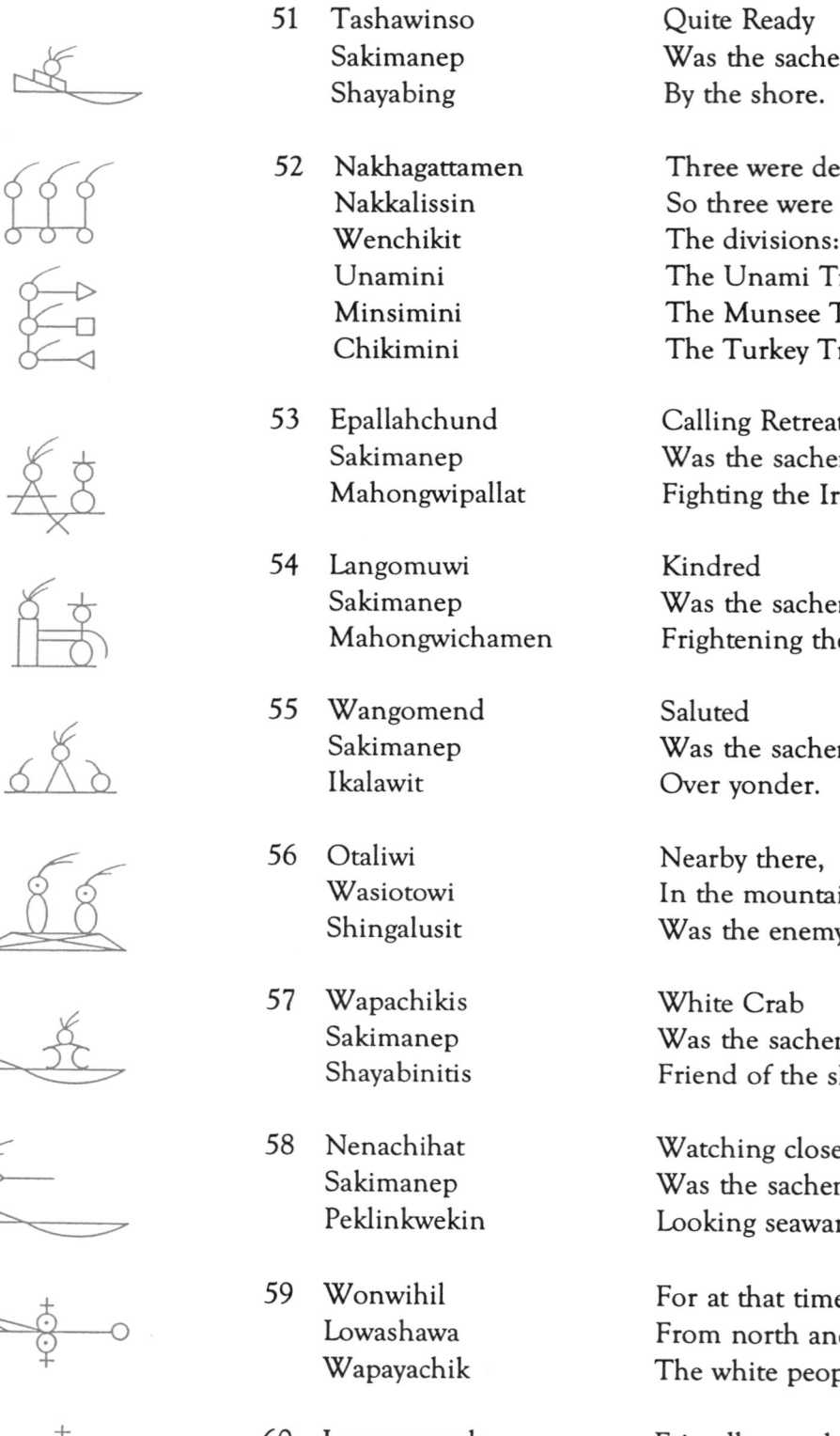

51	Tashawinso	Quite Ready
	Sakimanep	Was the sachem
	Shayabing	By the shore.

52	Nakhagattamen	Three were desired,
	Nakkalissin	So three were to be
	Wenchikit	The divisions:
	Unamini	The Unami Tribe,
	Minsimini	The Munsee Tribe,
	Chikimini	The Turkey Tribe.

53	Epallahchund	Calling Retreat
	Sakimanep	Was the sachem,
	Mahongwipallat	Fighting the Iroquois.

54	Langomuwi	Kindred
	Sakimanep	Was the sachem,
	Mahongwichamen	Frightening the Iroquois.

55	Wangomend	Saluted
	Sakimanep	Was the sachem,
	Ikalawit	Over yonder.

56	Otaliwi	Nearby there,
	Wasiotowi	In the mountains,
	Shingalusit	Was the enemy.

57	Wapachikis	White Crab
	Sakimanep	Was the sachem,
	Shayabinitis	Friend of the shore.

58	Nenachihat	Watching closely
	Sakimanep	Was the sachem,
	Peklinkwekin	Looking seaward.

59	Wonwihil	For at that time
	Lowashawa	From north and south,
	Wapayachik	The white people came.

60	Langomuwak	Friendly people,
	Kitohatewa	In great ships;
	Ewenikiktit?	Who are they?

Division and Invasion

Book V: verses 51 through 60

Great changes were in the air. The Lenni Lenape had grown so numerous that division was needed (V:51). Division is a natural consequence of growth, and more groups would have branched off if the Lenni Lenape's growth had not been cut off by the influx of the whites. The dividing lines were probably drawn according to geographical distribution—the upstream, midstream, and downstream regions of the Delaware River (V:52).[51]

Soon after this division, the Iroquoian Susquehannocks, also known as the Andaste, swept down from the north to conquer the Susquehanna Valley, cutting off the Lenni Lenape from their relatives to the west. The Lenni Lenape were forced to retreat (V:53) until they gathered enough of their Lenape relatives to stop the invaders (V:54). To the west in the Ohio country, the Lenape remained strong, but now an enemy force had been established between them and the Lenni Lenape, who maintained their presence along the East Coast.

Meanwhile, a powerful Lenape chief known as Powatan was uniting the tribes of Virginia under his sway, to counter the threats from the Susquehannocks to the north, the Siouans in the mountains to the south and west (V:56), and the approaching white colonists. He could be the "Saluted" mentioned in V:55. This was the situation that the English found when they arrived in Virginia to create the new settlement of Jamestown. One of them, Captain Samuel Argall, explored northward in 1610 and glimpsed what was then known as the River of the Lenape, dubbing the river the "Delaware" after the governor of Jamestown, Sir Thomas West, Lord de la Warr, so the people along its banks were included as the "Delaware Indians."[52] According to Heckewelder, they were at first uneasy about the name, but upon being told that it was the name of a great white chief, "As they are fond of being named after distinguished men, they were rather pleased, accepting it as a compliment."[53]

The Lenni Lenape or Delawares, as "Grandfathers" of the Lenape Family, were kept well informed of the progress of the various groups of European colonists arriving in Canada, New England, New York, Virginia, and Florida (V:58–59). Before long, the whites were sure to come to them, and at last, in 1638, a party of Swedish colonists came sailing up the river (V:60). The Wallam Olum, the Red Record, ends with the poignant question, "Who are they?"

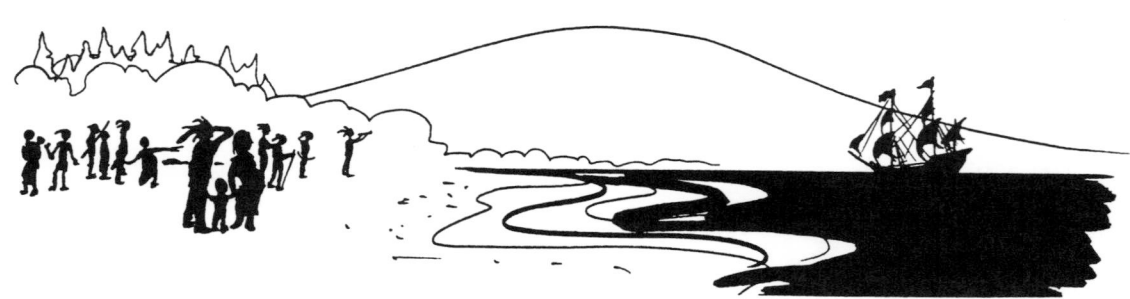

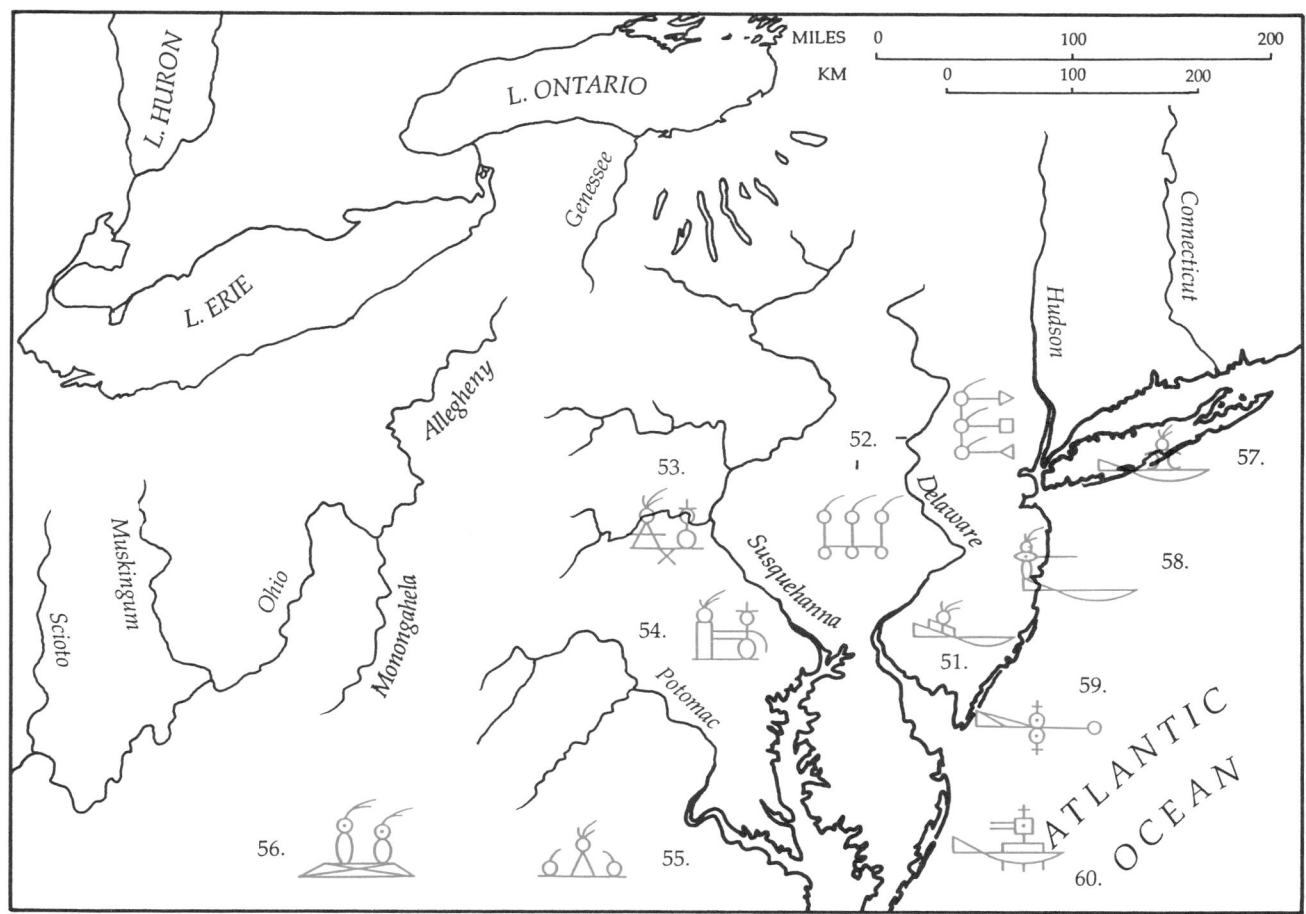

Figure 4.18. The map shows the location of the Lenape as revealed in verses **51** through **60** of Book V. The numbers on the map and in the box below refer to the verses in which the symbols and location clues appear.

Location Clues

51. This verse refers to the Delaware River homeland.

52. The Munsees (IV:29) were the northernmost Lenni Lenape division.

53. "Calling Retreat" refers to the loss of the Susquehanna Valley to the Iroquoian-speaking Susquehannocks.

54. This verse indicates a counterattack with the help of other Lenape tribes. The symbol refers to an overall region rather than to a specific place.

55. This verse may refer to the growing confederacy in Virginia.

56. Here, mention is made of enemies nearby. Siouan tribes such as the Monacans and the Tutelos remained strong in the Virginia mountains; there were also strong Iroquoian tribes such as the Cherokees to the southwest.

57. The symbol shows a crab at sea. The blue crab is a well-known edible swimming crab of the Atlantic coast.

58, 59, 60. As the years went by, the European colonies came closer and closer to the Lenni Lenape. By 1600, the French had moved into Canada, while the Spanish had come to Florida. By the 1620s, the English were becoming established in Virginia and New England, while the Dutch were preparing to move into New York. (See "The First Encounter" on page 140.)

The First Encounter

Fearlessly, the Lenape ambassador Mottschujinga, Little Grizzly Bear, went to meet them, nude in the ancient manner, carrying in one hand a black wampum belt containing a declaration of war, and in the other hand a Pipe of Peace, and waited for the strangers to make their choice.

> — *From the Lenape legend of their first encounter with the Iroquois.*[54]

In Arcadia we found a man who came to the shore to see what people we were: who stood hesitating and ready for flight. Watching us, he did not permit himself to be approached. He was handsome, nude, with hair fastened back in a knot, of olive color.

We were about [twenty in number] ashore and coaxing him he approached to within about two fathoms, showing a burning stick as if to offer us fire. And we made fire with gunpowder and flint and steel and he trembled all over with terror and we fired a shot.

> — *From Giovanni da Verrazano's report of the first landfall by Europeans in the territory of the Lenape, south of Delaware Bay.*[55]

Unless the Earth is one day invaded by aliens from another planet, we will never again know the feelings of surprise experienced by native people everywhere when the European explorers suddenly appeared from out of nowhere in their great ships. We can, however, understand the feelings by reading a description of the event in the Delawares' own words. The following account was recorded by Reverend John Heckewelder in 1762. It tells of the Delawares' first meeting with white people, when the Florentine explorer Giovanni da Verrazano sailed into what is now New York Harbor on April 17, 1524.

"*A great many seasons ago, some men of our nation, who were out at a place where the sea widens, espied, far away on the bosom of the Sea, a very large creature floating on the water. It was such an object as they had never seen before. Fear of this creature immediately filling their bosoms, they hastily returned to the shore. Having apprised their countrymen of what they had seen, they pressed them to accompany them, and make further discoveries of its nature and its purpose. Launching their canoes, they hurried out together,* and saw with increased astonishment the wonderful object which was approaching. Their conjectures were very various as to what it was; some believed it to be a great fish, or animal; while others were of the opinion that it was a very big house floating on the Sea. They were not long in concluding that this wonderful and mysterious object was moving towards the land, and they also saw that it was endued with life. Deeming it proper to inform all their brethren, to whom intelligence could be conveyed, of what was coming, that they might be on their guard, they dispatched swift runners and fast rowers in every direction, to the east, west and north, to carry the news to the scattered chiefs and tribes, that they might gather their warriors together, and prepare to combat, if need were, the strange creature. Soon, the chiefs and warriors of the neighboring tribes were collected in great numbers at that part of the shore which the strange creature was clearly approaching. It soon came so near that they were able to make it out to be a large moving house, in which, as they supposed, the Great Spirit himself was present, and coming to visit them.

"Wishing to receive him in a manner which should mark their sense of his goodness to them and their fathers, to the giver of the corn, and the victory over their enemies, they deliberated in what manner that object could be best accomplished. The first thing was to provide plenty of meat for a sacrifice, and with this in view the best hunters were dispatched to the forest; in quest of those animals supposed to be most acceptable to the mighty guest. The women were desired to prepare the choicest stews and pottage in the best manner. All the relics and sculptured images were brought out, examined and put in order. As a grand dance was always supposed to be an agreeable entertainment to the Great Spirit, one was ordered, not only for his gratification, but that it might, with the aid of a sacrifice, appease him, if he were angry with them, and induce him to stay his hand, rather than slay them. The priests and shamans were called, and set to work to determine, if possible, what this remarkable event portended, and what the possible result might be. They came habited in their robes of magic, skins of black bears, with the head, nose, eyes, teeth as also the legs, with the long claws, appearing the same as when the animal lived. Some were frightfully painted, some had the skin of an owl drawn over their heads, some had a huge pair of buffalo horns upon the head and a large bushy tail projecting from behind, and some had snakes wreathed around their bodies. To them, and to the chiefs and wise men of the nation, the women and children, and the men of inferior note, were looking up for protection and advice. And now, filling up their gourds with water from the stump of a fallen cypress, they begin the work of incantation, by muttering over the magic water a charm that had hitherto been of potent influence, and *words that called upon many spirits to assist in effecting the wishes of the masters of the spell. But the spirits answered not, and the priests became so distracted with fears at the unusual deafness of those who had given them their power, that they increased the fever of apprehension they should have assisted to calm. The gourds, with the charmed water, fell from their hands, and although the dance was commenced with fervor and enthusiasm, still it was greatly confused and irregular.*

"While in this situation, those men in canoes who had approached nearest to the strange object returned, and declared that it was a great house painted of various colors, and crowded with human beings. They thought it certain that it was the Great Spirit, bringing them some gift which they did not possess before. Other messengers soon arrived, who had seen the inhabitants of the house, and made a report which did not lessen their wonder, fear, or curiosity. They told their friends that they were men of a different color from the Lenape, and differently dressed; they were as white as the skin of a plucked bird, and wore no skins; and one of them, who must be the Great Spirit himself, was dressed entirely in red. The great house, or whatever it was, continued to approach. While approaching, some one in it cried to them in a loud voice, and in a language which they could not understand, yet they shouted in reply, according to the custom of the Mohicans and the Lenape. Much frightened at the strange voices, and at the still stranger creature which floated towards them, many proposed to retreat to the hills for security; others opposed this, lest offence should be given their visitor, who would find them out and destroy them. At last, the great creature, which they now found to be a great canoe, stopped and at once the robes white as snow, which were spread over its numerous arms, fluttered in the winds like clouds in the season of ripe corn. Soon there were many of the strange men employed in gathering these robes into folds, in the same manner as skins are packed.

"Presently a canoe of smaller size approached the shore where the people sat, having in it the man who was dressed in red and many others. When he had landed, leaving his canoe with some of his men to guard it, he approached the Mohican and Lenape chiefs and warriors who were assembled in council, and had seated themselves in a circle, as is their custom when about to receive ambassadors and messengers of peace. The man in red walked fearlessly into the midst of them, and saluted them all with great kindness, taking a hand of each, which he shook very hard. The Mohicans and Lenape, on their part, testified their gladness, and their friendship, and their emotions of joy and satisfaction at their arrival, by loud shouts, and by rubbing their cheeks against those of thier new acquaintances, and by patting them on the back. Lost in admiration of the strangers, of their dress, so gay and dissimilar to

their own, their manners so unlike, their features so different, and their language so unknown, the Mohicans and the Lenape could do nothing but wonder and applaud. A large portion of their admiration, however, was reserved for the man who wore the red coat with its glittering embroidery, and who, they doubted not, was the Great Spirit. The curiosity of the people was expressed in a thousand different ways; the priests wondered whether the Great Spirit knew and recognized them as old acquaintances; the warriors, whether the men who accompanied him were fleet, and courageous as themselves; and the women were very curious to know if the men were like our own men, and loudly expressed their determination to ascertain the fact. All agreed in this, that whether beings of this world, or of the world of dreams, they must be treated with great kindness, and fed upon the choicest viands of the tribe.

"Meanwhile; a large hackhack, or gourd, was brought to the man in red by one of his servants, from which he poured an unknown liquor resembling rain-water, into a small clear cup of such an appearance as the people had never before seen. He drank the liquor from this cup, and filling it again, he handed it to the chief next to him. The chief received it, smelt to it, and passed it untasted to the chief sitting by him, who did the same, till it had been handled and smelt to by all the Mohicans and Lenape in the circle, while not one had tasted it. The man who took the cup was upon returning it to the supposed Manito in red; when the Bender of the Pine Bow, one of the bravest and stoutest warriors in the nation, rose and spoke to his brothers thus:

It is not right for us to return the cup with its contents untasted. It is handed to us by the Manito, that we may drink as he has done. To follow his example will be pleasing to him; it will show our confidence in him, and the courage which we have been told is highly valued by him. To return the cup with its contents untasted, will give him reason to think that we believe it to be the juice of the Poison-tree; it will provoke his anger and bring destruction upon us all. It is for the good of the nation that the contents of the cup should be swallowed, and, as no one else will do it, the Bender of the Pine Bow devotes himself to the killing draught. It is better that one man should perish than that a whole nation should be destroyed.

"The Bender of the Pine Bow then took the glass, and giving many instructions, and bidding a solemn farewell to his family and friends, resolutely drank its fearful contents. Every eye was fixed on the brave man, to see what effect the strange liquor would produce. Soon he began to stagger, to whine fearfully, to roll up the white of his eyes, to shout, and to act a *thousand other extravagancies. At last, he fell prostrate on the ground. His companions, supposing him dead, fell to bemoaning his fate, and his wife set up the death-howl; all thought him a martyr to his valor and his love for his nation. But the man in red only laughed at their grief, and by signs gave them to understand that he would rise again. He told them true; the chief awoke and declared to his friends that he had enjoyed, while apparently lifeless, the most delicious sensations, and that he had never before felt so happy as after he had drunk the cup. He asked the man in red for more; his wish was granted; the other people made the same request, and so was theirs; the whole assembly tasted the contents of the cup, and all became as mad and intoxicated as their leader. Soon was the entire camp a scene of noise and tumult, brawl and bloodshed.*

"Meanwhile, the man in red, alarmed by the unexpected effects of the liquor, and by a sudden storm which came blowing in from the sea, hurriedly took his leave, after distributing gifts, and promising to return in a year. This came to pass, but later more and more came, in overwhelming numbers, until we were driven from our homes. But we have always kept the memory of that first meeting, and in commemoration of it, the island where it took place was ever after called Manahachtanienk, which means 'the island where we all became intoxicated,' a name which the whites have corrupted into 'Manhattan.'"

From Heckewelder, Reverend John. "The Coming of Miquon," in *Traditions of the North American Indians*, Vol. II, ed. James Athearn Jones, 99–105.[56]

Part Three

The Strangers

Chapter Five

"We Now Know Who They Are"

After the European explorers came the European colonists. With the coming of the first colonists to the Delaware River around 1620, the Red Record ends. But the Delawares' story continues in the final section of the Rafinesque Manuscript, which contains a valuable native view of their later history.

This historical glimpse is called the "Fragment." It is written in English, with Delaware names included, roughly translated by someone named John Burns from a lost Delaware original. There is no indication of any symbols. Rafinesque did not publish any other details on how this section was recorded and translated, but the historical information it contains corresponds to colonial and American records. The language of the translation is rough and irregular, with a few cryptic explanations mixed in with the text. It seems to be a basic, objective record of the meaning of the Delaware words, without regard for niceties of English composition, in the same way that Rafinesque recorded the literal meanings of the words of the Red Record without attempting to string the meanings into a more readable flow. But the Delaware original of the Fragment can still be sensed: a passionate lecture by a Delaware person, knowledgeable about his people's past, about the leaders and events of their long struggle from 1620 to the 1820s, when this account, and the Red Record, were recorded.

From the first, the Delawares had found themselves caught between the white and Indian worlds, acting as a bridge for positive diplomacy and greater understanding, as well as a channel for rage and revenge. They paid a heavy price for their exposed position; the forces that created the United States would shatter the unity of the Delawares and scatter them throughout the country. But despite this, the survivors still managed to affect the history of the American frontier to a degree far out of proportion to their small numbers. And a core group among them continued to carry on Delaware traditions and remember how their nation had fallen.

The Fragment is made up of twenty numbered paragraphs of different lengths. It contains many references to people and events in the Delawares' history that deserve fuller explanation. On the following pages, each paragraph is presented, transcribed verbatim from a photocopy of the original Rafinesque Manuscript housed at the University of Pennsylvania library (see Figure 5.1). (Words that were underlined in the original manuscript are also underlined in the transcription that follows.) Below each transcribed paragraph, which appears in italics, is a commentary that serves to expand the account into a more understandable narrative.

The Fragment below begins with an answer to the question posed in the last verse of the Red Record: "Who are they?"

FRAGMENT

On the History of the Linapis since abt 1600, when the <u>Wallamolum</u> *closes.*

translated from the Linapi–By John Burns

1. Halas, halas! we know now who they are, these Wapsinis (White men) who then came out of the Sea to rob us of our land; starving wretches! with smiles they came, but soon became Snakes or foes.

"Halas!" The Wallam Olum ends happily, with the joy and satisfaction of finding a homeland and cautious optimism about the visitors who were beginning to appear. But instead of a bright future, the Delawares were hit by a holocaust. For example, 14 different epidemics appear to have struck them after 1633, reducing their population by 90 percent, to fewer than 3,000, by the year 1700.[1] The psychological effects of such a loss of

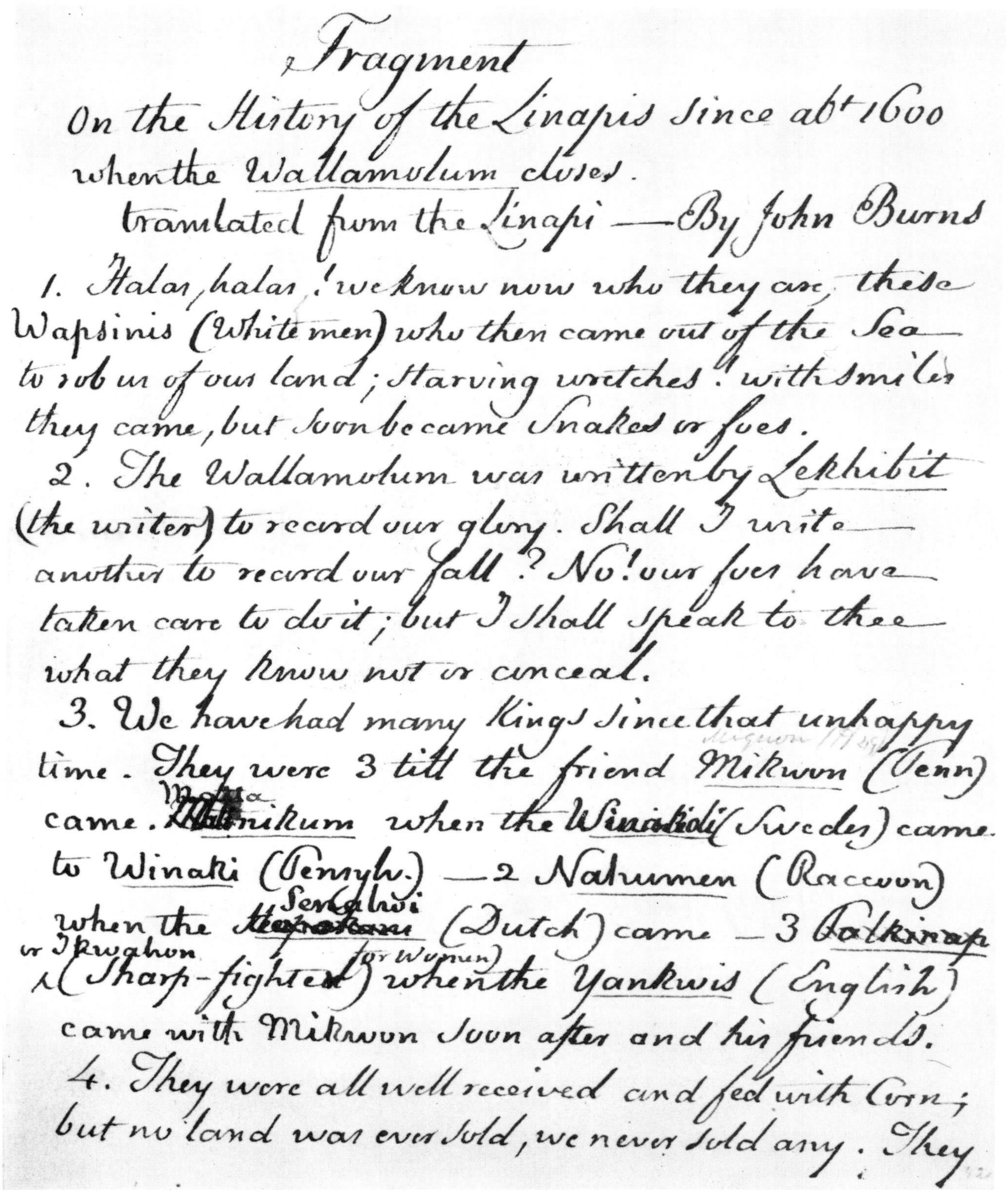

Fragment

On the History of the Linapis Since abt 1600
when the Wallamolum closes.

translated from the Linapi —— By John Burns

1. Halas, halas! we know now who they are, these
Wapsinis (White men) who then came out of the Sea
to rob us of our land; Starving wretches! with smiles
they came, but Soon became Snakes or foes.

2. The Wallamolum was written by Lekhibit
(the writer) to record our glory. Shall I write
another to record our fall? No! our foes have
taken care to do it; but I shall speak to thee
what they know not or conceal.

3. We have had many Kings Since that unhappy
time. They were 3 till the friend Mikwon (Penn)
came. Mikum when the Winakidi (Swedes) came.
to Winaki (Pennsylv.) — 2 Nahumen (Raccoon)
when the Senalwi (Dutch) came — 3 Palkinap
or Jkwahon
(Sharp-fighters) when the Yankwis (English)
came with Mikwon Soon after and his friends.

4. They were all well received and fed with Corn;
but no land was ever Sold, we never Sold any. They

Figure 5.1. A photograph of a page from the Rafinesque Manuscript shows the first page of the fragment written in Constantine Rafinesque's own hand.

family members, and the loss of the culture they embodied, can scarcely be imagined.

2. The Wallamolum was written by <u>Lekhibit</u> (the writer) to record our glory. Shall I write another to record our fall? No! our foes have taken care to do it; but I will speak to thee of what they know not or conceal.

"Lekhibit" probably refers to Lekhihitin, the Author, who is credited with helping to write the Red Record in the ancient past (see V:5). It is true that the foes of the Delawares took care to record their fall; almost no other American Indian tribe has been so fully documented over such a long period of time. But the Fragment still contains previously unknown material.

3. We have had many Kings since that unhappy time. There were 3 till the friend <u>Mikwon</u> (Penn) came. 1. <u>Mattanikum</u> when the <u>Winakoli</u> (Swedes) came to Winaki (Pennsylvania) – 2. <u>Nahumen</u> (Raccoon) when the [<u>Hopocani</u>] <u>Senalwi</u> (Dutch) came – 3. [<u>Palkinap</u>] or Ikwahon (Sharp-fighter for Women) when the <u>Yankwis</u> (English) came with Mikwon soon after and his friends.

The mention of "Kings" is a misnomer. The Delawares actually were a participatory democracy, so the presiding sachem was a first among equals, never a King, except in the misconceptions of the Europeans.

"Mikwon" (from *Miquin*, a feather, as in a quill pen) was the Delaware version of the name of William Penn. Penn was a leader of the Quakers, the Society of Friends, who was fondly remembered as a friend by the Delawares.

Mattanikum (from *Matta*, "no, not" and *niechin*, "to come down") is the first of the Delaware chiefs in the Fragment to be mentioned in European records. He was probably the sachem identified as "Mattahorn" by Peter Minuit when he acquired lands on behalf of Sweden in the 1640s, and by Peter Stuyvesant in later renegotiations for land for the Dutch in the 1650s.[2]

Swedish traders were the first to move into the Delawares' country, which here is called Winaki (Sassafras Country), an ancient name for Pennsylvania (see V:25). Under Captain "Big Guts" Prinze, the traders maintained a string of trading posts from 1638 to 1655, when the posts were captured by the Dutch.

Intensive fur hunting continued after the Dutch moved in. Here the Dutch are also called the Hopocani (pipe people, referring to their clay pipes). During this period, the Fragment says Nahumen (Raccoon) was chief. His name may be a misspelling; *nachenum* is "raccoon"; *nahimen*

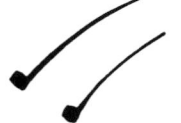

Clay pipes. The Dutch enjoyed smoking tobacco in clay pipes such as these.

is "to sail down the stream." The Dutch dominated the Delaware River fur trade from 1655 to 1664, when the English came and took over. The influential sachem identified as "Idquayhon" by Penn in several land sales late in the 1600s is probably the "Ikwahon" mentioned as the chief when the English came.[3] "Yankwis" may reflect the Lenape pronunciation of the word "English," which sounded like Yengees."[4] The English in the Delaware valley, under Governor Andros, at first made attempts to deal more fairly with the Delawares than did the Dutch, and tried to curb the sale of alcohol. Disease, alcohol, abuse by the Dutch colonists, and attacks by the Iroquois took a fearful toll on the Delawares during these years. The hunting grounds were becoming exhausted, and the Delawares, needing to travel to the fur-rich interior, agreed to pay tribute to the Iroquoian Susquehannocks.

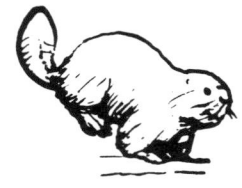

Beaver.
The fashion in Europe of wearing beaver furs drove trapping and settlement activity in America.

"Sharp-fighter for Women" may be a reference to the Delawares' being referred to as "women" by the Iroquois in the early 1700s. This may reflect their position as mediators for peace among the Lenape tribes and between the Lenape and the Europeans—in the Native American metaphor, peace negotiators would be "women" as opposed to "warriors." The Iroquois, however, claimed that the Delawares had been conquered and forced to become non-combatants or "women." In either case, the Delawares' position was eventually taken as an excuse for their abuse by both the Iroquois and the English.[5]

Then William Penn, whom the Delawares called Mikwon, took over the Pennsylvania territory as a refuge for the Quakers and instituted a policy of fair dealings with the Delawares, a policy based on respect and equal justice.

4. They were all well received and fed with Corn; but no land was ever sold, we never sold any. They were allowed to live with us, to build houses and plant Corn, as our friends and allies. Because they were hungry, and thought Children of Sunland and not Snakes or children of Snakes.

The generous hospitality of the Delawares and their Lenape relatives helped keep European colonies and trading posts alive. "Children of Sunland" reflects the extra consideration given to the Europeans because of the initial Lenape belief that the people from out of the East, their sacred direction, were somehow divine. But when the colonists began to demand the food as their right, in the form of taxes, trouble ensued.

Despite the amicable personal relations between the Delawares and Penn, their society and English society were so fundamentally different that conflict was almost inevitable. For example, the Fragment asserts that "no land was ever sold," and there is still debate over whether land sales in the usual sense did occur.[6] It is clear from the initial sales documents that indeed there was a misunderstanding about the idea of land sales in the European sense, which was and still is an alien idea to Native Americans. It was not thought that a sale entitled one to fence in and absolutely exclude others, especially the original inhabitants, from all use rights. This would have been equivalent to a house guest's claiming the deed to a house because of a host's courteous statement, "My house is your house." The documents also reveal that the first land sales were negotiated between Europeans and Delaware individuals or families. As the Delawares gained more sophistication in the procedure, they worked to elevate the negotiations from sales between individuals to treaties between nations, helping to establish a precedent that has been followed ever since.

5. And they were traders, bringing fine new tools and weapons and cloth and beads, for which we exchanged Skins and wampuns. And we liked them and their things because we thought they were good, and made by Children of Sunland.

The first European settlements were trading posts. Any Delaware trading common wampum beads and beaver furs for rare and precious metal utensils and weapons must have felt he was getting the best of the bargain. European goods were in such demand among other tribes farther inland that Delaware traders could make great profits as middlemen. But these riches came at an increasing price. The demand for furs forced the Delawares to hunt more and more until the beaver were gone from their territory, and the only way to obtain furs was from the dangerous Iroquoian tribes inland.

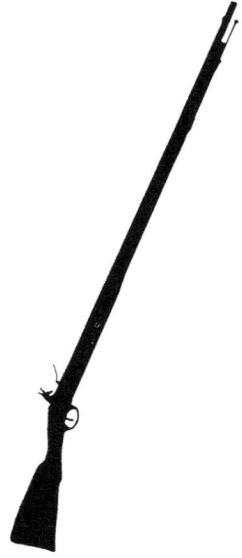

Flintlock guns. The British "brown Bess" musket shown here is unique; since each gun was made from custom-made parts, no two were alike.

6. But alas they brought also Fireguns & Fire Water, which burned & killed. Also baubles & trinkets of no use: since we had better ones.

Guns and rum created destructive dependencies that demoralized and destroyed the native culture. Guns made hunting easier, but they also made the hunter dependent on the trader for gunpowder and lead. Alcohol was used quite consciously by unscrupulous whites to seduce, confuse, and debauch native people so they could be cheated out of their goods, their land, and their rights.

The Delawares were also cheated by trade goods of inferior quality—"baubles and trinkets of no use" and not the equal of native goods made for the same purpose. Traders and treaty negotiators would also give out those goods that they had at hand, rather than goods that the Indians may have actually needed. Leaders of recurrent native religious revivals were continually urging the Indians to give up the white man's goods and revive their ancient crafts.

7. And after <u>Mikwon</u> came the children of <u>Dolojo Sakima</u> (King George) who said more land more land we must have, and no limits could be put to their steps and increase.

After their good experiences with William Penn, the Delawares were confronted by his land-hungry successors. "Dolojo Sakima" is the Delaware rendition of the name of King George of England, used generically in the Fragment for George I, George II, and George III. The English demand "more land more land we must have" became a constant refrain from here on.

To get away from the growing English settlements, the Delawares gradually moved up the Delaware River. The pressure for land sales climaxed when the heirs of William Penn, in need of money, decided to defraud the Delawares with the notorious "Walking Purchase." In 1735, Penn's heirs pressured the Delawares into agreeing to sell land extending "as far as a man can walk in a day and a half" in a specified direction. The heirs then made a trail through the forest into the heart of the remaining Delaware territory, and sent runners along this pre-cut path to grab as much land as they could. One of the runners suffered permanent damage from his exertions. Surveying lines then were drawn from the farthest point reached so as to claim the remaining Delaware territory, and the Iroquois were called in to help force the Delawares to leave.[7] The shock of the fraud soured relations between the Delawares and the English, and convinced most of the Delawares to abandon their homeland for lands in the Susquehanna Valley and farther west in Ohio.

8. But in the North were the children of <u>Lowi-Sakima</u> (King Louis) and they were our good friends, allies of our allies, foes of our foes; yet Dolojo always wanted to war with them.

The subjects of King Louis were the French traders and settlers of Canada, the Great Lakes, and the Mississippi Valley. While the English cultivated a friendship with the Iroquois of the Six Nations, the enemies of the Delawares, the French were friends with the Delawares' allies—the Wyandots, an Iroquoian tribe the Delawares called the Talamatans, and the Lenape tribes of Canada and the Midwest. In general, the English were more interested in getting Native Americans' land, while the French were more interested in enlisting them to hunt for furs. France and England were bitter rivals for colonial territories in America and elsewhere in the world.

> *9. We had 3 Kings after Mikwon. <u>Skalichi</u> (or Last Tamanend), 2 <u>Sassunam Wikwikhon</u> (Our Uncle Builder) and 3 <u>Tatami</u> (Beaver Taker). This last was killed by a <u>Yankwako</u> English Snake, and we vowed revenge.*

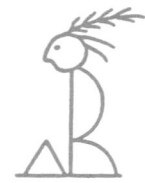

Symbol for Tamanend. Tamenend the First, a great peacemaker, is represented by this symbol in the Red Record.

The first of the "3 Kings," Skalichi, was recorded as "Skalitchy" in land sale documents of the time, and also as "Tamanend." He would have been Tamanend the Third, taking into account the two mentioned previously in the Red Record (see IV:35–36 and V:32). He and other sachems negotiated several famous land sales with William Penn around 1683, during what may have been the most fruitful period of White-Indian relations. Later, Tamanend was adopted in the nineteenth century as the "patron saint of America" by the St. Tammany Society, a fraternal organization that went on to have a darker history as Tammany Hall.[8]

The second King was "Sassunam Wikwikhon." This refers to Sassoonan, who was also known as "Olumapies," which denotes a role as record-keeper like Olumapi in the Red Record (see IV:23). Sassoonan was set up as "King of the Delawares" by the corrupt successors of William Penn in the 1730s to simplify their land negotiations. Unfortunately, he was a weak-willed man, who was no more than a puppet ruler. He was so addicted to drink that he even sold off the wampum records of past treaties in exchange for rum. During his time, the Delawares were forced to give up the last of their ancient homeland along the Delaware River. Sassoonan tried to set up a refugee center for the Delawares and their relatives in the Lebanon Valley, but was forced in the end to sell it as well.[9]

The identification of the third King, "Tatami" (Beaver Taker), is unclear. The Tatamy family from the Munsie country to the north moved down to be among the leaders of the refugees living in the remaining Delaware land between the Forks of the Delaware. The chief leader of the Delawares of the Fork was Nutimus (Fish Spearer), a contemporary of Sassoonan, who had a different territory. After Nutimus and his people were driven out by the notorious "Walking Purchase," they went to settle on the Susquehanna on lands claimed by the Iroquois. These lands had been given to the Delawares and other Lenape refugees under Iroquois "protection" as a buffer against further westward expansion by the whites. After Sassoonan died in 1747, there was no one immediately available to succeed him who had the approval of the Delawares as well as their new overlords, the Pennsylvania authorities and the Iroquois Six Nations. Finally the choice devolved on two brothers in the line of succession from Sassoonan—the quiet Tamaqua (Beaver), who acted as the peace chief and who might be the "Beaver Taker" referred to here, and the fiery Shingas (Marshy Ground) who became the war chief, reasserting the power of the

Delawares. His later exploits against settlers during the French and Indian War would earn him the nickname of "Shingas, the Terrible."

10. Netawatwis (first renewed being) became king of all the Nations in the West, again at <u>Talligewink</u> (Ohio) on the R. Cayahaga, with our old allies the Talamatans (Hurons or Guyandots) and calls all from the East.

"Netawatwis," more commonly spelled $Netawatwees" (Skilled Advisor), was the distinguished chief of the Delawares in the West, and had great influence among the Delawares and their allies from the late 1750s until the beginning of the Revolutionary War. Under him, the Delawares regrouped in the Ohio Valley and were allowed by their old allies the Talamatans or Wyandots to reoccupy the Talega country they had lived in long before, as described in the Red Record. In Ohio, the Delaware refugees from Pennsylvania as well as Lenape survivors from New Jersey, New York, and New England found a safe haven. The new Delaware territories were centered in eastern Ohio, from the Cayahoga River to the north to the Muskingum River to the south, where the Delaware capital of Coshocton stood.

Netawatwees, who as a boy had witnessed the signing of treaties with William Penn, died in 1776 at the age of ninety-nine, after lighting the council fire and opening deliberations for the first United States-Indian peace treaty.

First United States flag. This flag of the United States dates from the Revolutionary era.

11. But Tadescung was king at the East at Mahoning and bribed by the Yankwis; there he was burned in his house, and many of our people massacred at Hickory (Lancaster) by the Land robbers. Yankwis.

"Tadescung" refers to Teedyuscung (He Who Makes the Earth Tremble), an astute diplomat and champion of his people who was also known as "Honest John" Harris. He had been converted to Christianity by the pacifist Moravian missionaries, who were setting up model communities dedicated to order, sobriety, and justice for the Indians on the frontier.

Teedyuscung acted as the leader of the remaining Delawares in the Susquehanna Valley, who were centered at Wyoming (here spelled "Mahoning") where he tried to remain neutral after the outbreak of the French and Indian War in 1755. But the indifference of the English, plus the success of Shingas' Delawares from Ohio in their attacks upon English settlements, caused Teedyuscung to also go on the warpath. Afterwards, he presided over the re-establishment of peace along the Susquehanna. Then he became embroiled in English politics, as the

Quakers pushed him to complain about the Walking Purchase to embarrass the Pennsylvania authorities. The Pennsylvania authorities, however, plied Teedyuscung with gifts and fair promises, and these, plus concern about the vulnerability of his people, persuaded him to desist. To show their appreciation, the authorities built cabins for him and the other Delawares, but would not grant his pleas for title to his own land. A Connecticut land company staked a claim to the Susquehanna, and sent a flood of trespassers to simply take over. Teedyuscung's protests were in vain, and on the evening of April 19, 1763, his cabin was set afire, burning him to death, and the Delaware town of Wyoming was turned to ashes.[10]

After the death of Teedyuscung, no place was allowed for the Delawares in Pennsylvania. In December 1763, the so-called Paxton Boys, out of hatred of the Indians and a desire to avenge the victims of Indian attacks, committed two massacres of peaceful, unarmed Conestoga Indian men, women, and children living in Lancaster. Subsequently, they tried to massacre 140 pacifist Delaware Moravian converts, who had to be locked in a dungeon in Philadelphia for safety. The government added its backing to the movement by offering large bounties for Delaware scalps, from whatever source.

12. Then we joined our friend Lowi in war against the Yankwis; but they were strong and took Lowanaki (North land) from Lowi, and came to us in Talegawink when peace was made: and we called them Bigknives, Kichikani.

The Delawares were forced by many factors to "join our friend Lowi" and take the French side in the French and Indian War. A contemptuous dismissal of a Delaware offer of assistance to the English General Braddock before his disastrous defeat in 1755 was certainly a factor. Other determining factors included the English designs on owning the Ohio valley and filling it with settlers, the domination of French traders in the Ohio valley, and the Delawares' desire to reassert their power as warriors and gain revenge for past injuries by the English. Delaware war parties spread terror across the frontier as far east as New Jersey. But when French supplies began to run out, the Ohio Delawares proposed peace, if the English could guarantee that no families would be allowed to settle west of the Alleghenies. The English, anxious to pass through Delaware lands to attack the French, agreed, and the peace was made. English forces then passed through the Delaware lands and late in 1758 seized the strategic forks of the Ohio, where they began construction of the massive Fort Pitt. This changed the balance of power on the frontier and led to the French loss of Canada and the end of the war early in

1763. But the English forces did not withdraw, declaring that they would stay to "protect" the Indians, and it became obvious that settlers would soon be coming to the Ohio valley.

Desperately, the Delawares in Ohio, inspired by Neolin, the Delaware Prophet, spread the word that to preserve their homes, they must restore their ancient way of life and strike the English. Their rallying cry was, "Our brethren, let us die together, since the design of the English is to destroy us. We are dead one way or the other." Pontiac, an Ottawa war captain from Michigan, adopted this message and gathered the tribes of the Midwest together to attack. They swept eastward across the frontier and captured all the English outposts except Fort Pitt, Detroit, and Niagara, which they besieged. By June, it looked as if the tribes would succeed. But the Delawares and Shawnees besieging Fort Pitt were struck with smallpox. The disease had been spread by infected blankets given to them during truce negotiations in accordance with instructions from General Amhearst to "extirpate this execrable race."[11] At the end of the summer, the besiegers were starving and running low on ammunition, and the siege was finally broken by a force led by the Swiss mercenary Colonel Henry Bouquet.

Bouquet followed up his success with an unprecedented attack deep into the Ohio territory, where he seized the important Delaware town of Coshocton at the forks of the Muskingum. Exhausted by war, the Delawares had no choice but to make peace and give up their hundreds of captives. Many of these white captives, however, did not want to leave their Indian families, and they had to be taken back under armed guard. As the returning captives were streaming eastward, the last of the Delawares in Pennsylvania were being forced westward. Their Iroquois overlords had given the Susquehanna valley to the English. Aside from two tiny reservations in Massachusetts and southern New Jersey, there were now no Delawares left east of Ohio.

The Treaty of Fort Stanwix in 1768 reserved for the Indians the lands west of the Alleghenies and north of the Ohio River. But the land south of the Ohio, including most of the hunting preserve of Kentucky, was given to the English by the Iroquois, who did not own it in the first place. "Bigknives, Kitchikani" (describing swords) was a name particularly applied to the Virginians, who were especially aggressive in laying claim to land in Kentucky and elsewhere in the Ohio Valley. Fights in Kentucky between the Shawnee and the encroaching Virginians turned the area into what became known as "the dark and bloody ground."

13. Then Alimi (Whiteyes) and Gelelenund (Buck-killer) were chiefs, and all the Nations near us were allies under us or our grandchildren again. When the Eastern fires began to resist Dolojo, they said we should be another fire with them.

The reference to "Alimi" is unclear. There was a blind Munsie sachem in Ohio named "Allemewi" who was converted by the incoming Moravian missionaries and renamed "Solomon." The Moravian missionaries, from the German United Brethren, did much to bring needed farming, blacksmithing, animal husbandry, and other skills to the Delawares, and with the sponsorship of the aging Netawatwees, the Christian and non-Christian Delawares and their relatives were united in towns along the Tuscarawas in Ohio. There they lived peacefully until the outbreak of the American Revolution.

"Gelelenund" refers to Gelelemend (Leader), Netawatwees' grandson, also known as Captain John Killbuck, Jr. He was more sympathetic to the Moravians than was his father, John Killbuck, Sr., Netawatwees' son. Between them, they represented the traditionalist and Christian divisions among the Delawares.

"Whiteyes" is the more important name mentioned here. It refers to White Eyes, whose usual Delaware name was "Coquetakeghton" (That Which Is Near the Head). This eloquent and visionary sachem persuaded the Delawares in 1774 not to assist the Shawnees in Kentucky in what became known as Lord Dunmore's War. White Eyes convinced the Delawares that their long-term interests would be served by cooperating with the English instead of opposing them.

Gathered together again under Netawatwees and his elected successor, White Eyes, the surviving Delawares, now numbering around 3,000 in total, found a new sense of themselves that made them influential far beyond their numbers. They were valued participants in events throughout the frontier. As the Fragment puts it, "all the Nations near us were allies under us or our granchildren again." The influence of the Delawares can also be seen in the line, "When the Eastern Fires . . . said we should be another fire with them," which refers to one of the most fascinating and little-known chapters in the history of the frontier.

At the outbreak of the American Revolution, the talented and energetic George Morgan was appointed by the Continental Congress as an ambassador to go to the Delawares and the other Indian nations of the West to encourage them to remain neutral instead of joining the British to win vengeance against the colonists. That he succeeded in this, despite long odds, was due in large part to the help he received from his friend White Eyes, who traveled among many tribes and also brought his message of friendship to the Americans in Philadelphia in an address to the Continental Congress. As the Moravian missionary Reverend David Zeisberger commented, "If the Delawares had taken part against the Americans in the present war, America would have had terrible experiences; for the neutrality of the Delawares kept all the many nations that are their grandchildren neutral also, except the Shawanese, who are no longer in close union with their grandfathers."[12]

The outcome of Morgan's efforts was the first treaty conference between the Americans and the Indian nations. Led by the Delawares, the conference took place in the American fortress at Fort Pitt in 1776. (The details of this conference and the events leading up to it have only recently been published.[13]) At Morgan's suggestion, White Eyes worked hard to gather the scattered Delawares together around Coshocton in Ohio for their own protection, and so that some elements would not go off to the war on their own. His vision was that the Delawares would become the core of a nation of Christian, self-sufficient Indians, living unmolested in their own territory in the Midwest. As the Revolutionary War went on, the Delawares, by now split into pro-English and pro-American factions, were facing overwhelming pressure to choose sides. In a gamble, the leaders of the Delawares, led by White Eyes, made a treaty with American representatives on September 17, 1778, wherein it was agreed to form a confederation headed by the Delawares; this confederation could become the fourteenth state of the Union. However, the treaty had been misrepresented to the Delaware leaders, for it was intended to involve the Delawares heavily on the side of the Americans.[14] An expedition was being formed to attack the British at Detroit, and the Americans promised to build a fort near Coshocton to protect the Delawares from retaliation if they could have guides and safe passage through the Delaware territories. White Eyes, who was made a lieutenant colonel in the American forces, offered to be their guide.

14. But they killed [Gelelemund] our chiefs <u>Unamiwi</u> (turtling) & our brothers on Muskingum, and Hopokan of the Wolf tribe was made king and made War on the Kichikani Yankwis rather choosing Dolojo for ally as he was so Strong.

Soon after the expedition set out to attack the British at Detroit, the news was spread that White Eyes had died of smallpox. The truth, which was kept secret for many years, was that the Americans had treacherously murdered him. The American expedition White Eyes had tried to lead was bungled, and the Americans withdrew, leaving the Delawares exposed to the angered English and their Indian allies.

In addition to White Eyes, the promising young direct heir to Netawatwees was murdered. He was slain in 1782 by white settlers in Pennsylvania, who stole the bag containing the Delawares' wampum records and deeds since the time of William Penn.[15] These two deaths deprived the Unami Turtle clan, which had acted as the senior branch of government since Netawatwees, of its most qualified leaders.

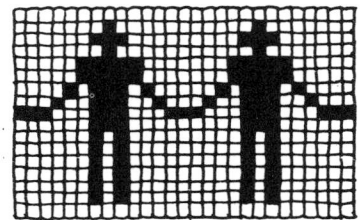

Wampum design. This design in a wampum treaty belt shows figures holding hands.

The Delawares were still being forced to choose sides in the Revolution. Fed up with the empty promises and empty hands of the Americans and under pressure to join with their other Indian allies, a strong faction led by White Eyes' pro-British rival, identified here as "Hopokan of the Wolf Tribe," took control of the Delaware Tribal Council and accepted British support in return for attacks on the Americans. Delaware war parties led by Hopokan, better known as Captain Pipe, and the warrior Buckonga-helas (One Whose Movements Are Certain) soon had a devastating impact across the frontier.[16] These attacks, however, unleashed American reprisals. The worst of these occurred in March 1782 deep in Delaware country in Ohio. A force of American frontiersmen led by Lieutenant Colonel Williamson cold-bloodedly massacred at least ninety unarmed, pacifist Delaware Moravian converts at Gnadenhutten (Huts of Grace) and burned it and other neighboring Moravian mission towns to the ground.[17]

15. But the Eastern fires were Stronger; they did not take Lowanaki, but became free from Dolojo. We went to Wapahani (White R.) to be farther from them; but they follow every where & we made War on them, till they sent <u>*Makhiakho*</u> *(Black Snake, Genl. Wayne) who made strong war.*

After their victory at Yorktown, the Americans announced that the United States, as a new nation, was not bound by the settlement limits agreed to by the British. A confederacy of thirty-five tribes, including the Delawares, banded together with the support of the British in Canada to resist the incoming settlers. The Delawares by this time were beginning to accept the invitation of their Lenape relatives the Miamis to settle on Miami lands along the White River between present-day Muncie and Indianapolis in Indiana.

Settlers were soon coming near even these areas, and the united tribes, including Delaware warriors under Buckongahelas, fought back under the leadership of the Miami war chief Little Turtle, a military genius whose mother was a Mohican. American armies sent against the united Lenape tribes went down to defeat again and again—first General Harmer's army in 1790, then Governor St. Clair's army in 1791—in the greatest victories ever won by Indian armies in American history.

Finally, in 1794, a specially trained force under General "Mad" Anthony Wayne, here called Makhiakho (Black Snake) marched into what is now Indiana. Little Turtle urged that negotiations be opened to conclude a peace, but he was overruled and deposed. Wayne then caught the outnumbered and undersupplied Lenape forces and crushed them in a forest that had been wrecked by a tornado. This became known as the Battle of Fallen Timbers.

16. We made peace and settle limits, and our next King was Hakhing-pomskan (hard walker) who was good, and peaceful. He would not join our Brothers Shawanis & Ottawas nor Dolojo in the new war.

The Delawares made peace and settlement limits the next year, in 1795, with the Treaty of Greenville, which opened the territory of Ohio to white settlers. In return, the tribes were guaranteed lands in most of the rest of what was then called the Northwest Territory.[18]

"Hakhing-Pomskan" (Hard Walker), also known as Hockingpomska, was the next leader from the Wolf Clan.[19] Tetepachsit, from the Turtle clan, was actually the nominal head of the Delawares at this time; omission of his name may indicate that the author of the Fragment was a Wolf. Like his friend the warrior Buckongahelas, Hockingpomska kept the vow he had made at Greenville never again to take up arms against the Americans, but he also followed the advice in Buckongahelas' last words: "Never trust a white man."

By this time, the Indians of the White River region wanted to have as little to do with white people as possible. They shunned missionaries and the land-hungry Governor William Henry Harrison, and listened attentively to the nativist revival message of Tenskwatawa (The Open Door), better known as the Shawnee Prophet. With his accusations of witchcraft, the Prophet instigated the murder of Tetepachsit, the Delaware chief, who was tomahawked and burned to death in front of his people. Such tactics led the Delawares to vote against joining the Prophet's charismatic brother Tecumseh in his attempt to unite the tribes to keep the Americans at bay. Harrison's army was thus able to defeat the Prophet's forces decisively in 1811 at Tippecanoe. Exploiting this victory would later win Harrison the Presidency, but he would die of an illness caught on Inauguration Day.

Another opportunity for Tecumseh to strike at the Americans was soon at hand. The War of 1812 broke out, and Tecumseh, made a brigadier general by the British in Canada, enlisted many of the tribes, including the Delawares' hosts the Miamis, to fight for the British cause. Despite enormous pressure, the Delawares maintained their neutrality, and several Delawares performed valuable services for the Americans.

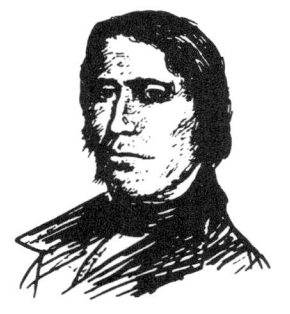

Portrait of Tecumseh. The great Indian resistance leader, Tecumseh, died in battle against the Americans in 1813.

17. After the last peace, the Yankwis came in crowds all around us, and they want again our lands of Wapahani: it was useless to resist, because they are getting Stronger and Stronger, by increasing their United Fires.

After the War of 1812, the United States government moved to extinguish, as quickly as possible, Indian title to lands east of the Mississippi such as Delaware lands along the Wapahani (White River).

The tribes were induced through payments to exchange their lands in the East for lands of supposedly equal worth west of the Mississippi. This was known as the Removal Policy. The pressure to remove the Indians quickly became intense because the Indians' lands were the best cleared, and thus were the ones settlers wanted most. By 1816, there were so many settlers in Indiana that it was admitted to the Union as a state, becoming another of the "United Fires," and the Delawares could see that their days in Indiana were numbered.

18. Kithtitkund & Lapanibi (White Water) were the chiefs of our 2 tribes, when we resolved to exchange our lands and return at last beyond the Masispek (muddy water or Mississippi) near to our Ancient Seat.

There were two major divisions of the Delawares at this time. The chief of one was Kithtitkund or Kikthawenund (Creaking Boughs), also known as Chief William Anderson. This Turkey clan chief, whose influence in Delaware affairs had been felt as early as the 1790s, became chief after the death of Tetapachsit at the hands of the Shawnee Prophet. Anderson had a white father, but through his mother's connections and his own temperament, he was fully a part of the Delaware nation, in which he was much admired.[20]

The chief of the other division was Lapanibi (White Water), more properly "Lapinihile" (Must Be Killed Twice), also known as Big Bear.[21] He and Chief Anderson were the leaders of the Delawares when they reluctantly accepted the offers of the government in the Treaty of Saint Marys in 1818, and agreed to remove to lands of equal worth west of the Mississippi.

These lands are described here as "near to our Ancient Seat," a reference to the ancient locations for the Lenni Lenape described in the Red Record, which makes it clear that long ago they lived west of the Mississippi (see IV:48–51).

19. We shall be near our foes the <u>Wakon</u> (Ozages) but they are better than the <u>Yankwiakon</u> (English Snakers) who want to possess the whole Big Island.

The displacement of the many Indian nations of the East into the West was bound to have a disruptive effect both on the people already living in the West and on the migrants from the East. For the first time, the Delawares would be living in territories not controlled by their Lenape relatives, such as the Miamis, or by their friends, such as the Wyandots. They would have to find and claim homes in a hostile wilderness, facing formidable enemies such as the Osage. But at least their foes would be

Indians like themselves in a place outside of the lies and broken promises of the United States. The bitter claim here that the Americans wanted to "possess the whole Big Island" must have seemed far-fetched in the 1820s, but would later prove prophetic. Within twenty-five years, the United States would declare war on Mexico in order to fulfill its "Manifest Destiny" to extend from the Atlantic to the Pacific.

20. Shall we be free and happy there? at the New Wapahani, We want rest and peace and Wisdom.

The Delawares began their move into the West. Their previous homes had been along the White River in Indiana, where Dr. Ward was given the Red Record in 1820. Here "the New Wapahani" refers to the Delawares' destination, the James Fork of the White River in Missouri. The westward trek of the Delawares was long and painful. By 1821, they had all crossed the Mississippi into the West, where they hoped to find a home where they would be left alone.

Like the Red Record, the Fragment ends with a question, as the Delawares looked into an uncertain future with cautious hope.

Chapter Six

Homes in Exile

D ecimated by disease, cheated out of their lands, swamped by an
alien culture, defeated in war, and forced into exile, the Delawares
nevertheless survived, to leave an indelible mark on history.

The exodus of the Delawares out of the East was part of the larger
eviction of the tribes westward throughout the 1820s and '30s most
famously represented by the Cherokees' "Trail of Tears." At the time, the
area beyond the Mississippi was almost unknown, and was not thought
fit for settlement; the Great Plains were called the Great American Desert.
It was thought that this region would remain wilderness, outside the
limits of the United States, allowing the tribes, both the native and the
displaced ones, to live there undisturbed. This was the earliest phase of
the western frontier; as pioneers, the Delawares were among the first—and
among the most prominent—of the Eastern tribes in this, the Wildest
West.

Their stormy history left the Delawares torn into several communities.
The main body totaling around 1,300 had left lands on the White River
in Indiana and near Piqua in Ohio, crossed the Mississippi, and relocated
on the James Fork of the White River in Missouri by the end of 1821.

One Delaware group was already in Missouri, having removed themselves beginning in 1789 to go west to live in what were then Spanish lands near Cape Girardeau. While some of these so-called "Absentee" Delawares joined the main body when it arrived, about 700 continued south, renouncing money promised by government treaties in order to live a life of freedom in territories not yet within the United States. They took up lands in East Texas at the invitation of the Mexican government, and befriended the local tribes such as the Caddo Confederacy and the free tribes of the plains to the north. In Canada, there were four communities of Delaware refugees and their close relatives, totaling about 1,000 souls, who had at various times come north from New York, Pennsylvania, and Indiana. The most prominent community, made up of Moravian Christians, lived in towns along the Thames River near Fairfield in Ontario. In Wisconsin, former mission Delawares with their relatives formed a small but cohesive group called the Stockbridge-Munsies, who were originally from Stockbridge, Massachusetts, and included the New Jersey Brothertons.

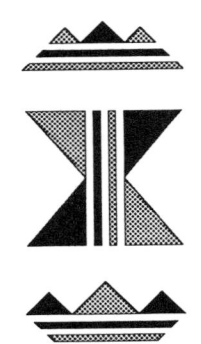

Delaware design. This Delaware design is based on one recorded by Frank Speck.

In southeastern Missouri, the main body of the Delawares along with their Lenape relatives the Shawnee, Kickapoo, Piankashaw, Peoria, and Wea, as well as their Iroquoian friends the Cherokees, occupied a wooded, hilly country near the Ozarks. They had had trouble there almost from the first. The land, though fertile, was subject to floods; crop after crop was washed out and lost. There was almost no game; the Delaware hunters had to go far afield, where they soon ran into murderous conflict with the Siouan-speaking Osages who resented their presence.

Chief William Anderson, the elderly leader of the Delawares, struggled to find a better home for his people. He wanted to see them settled in a land they could call their own before he died. Delaware hunters explored the woodlands bordering the prairie, from East Texas northward. In 1830, they found what they wanted. The Delawares agreed to move to a home farther west, a large reservation of over two million acres set aside for them in northeastern Kansas, which was then unorganized territory.

Delaware design. This Delaware design is based on one recorded by Frank Speck.

Here, the Delawares had a much happier time. The government aid and cash annuities they had won in various treaties over the years now added up to significant amounts. Missionaries organized schools for Delaware children. Their new homeland—which extended from the mouth of the Kansas River northward almost to Fort Leavenworth and westward for 200 miles toward the buffalo country on the Great Plains—was fertile, with timber and good farmland. Soon the Delaware families were building themselves comfortable houses, farms, and ranches; hunting far across the Plains to the west, and south through the woodlands and prairies to their Absentee Delaware relatives in Texas.

The author Washington Irving, on a visit to the Great Plains in 1832, noted in his journal that among the tribes: "the bravest and finest race is the Delawares. They are called the [grand]*fathers*—all the others give them preference . . . all their equipments of the best—their camp kettles of brass. They are clean, neat, civil, generously obliging, light hearted, gay, fearless—go to the Rocky Mountains in bands of 20 men—have frequent skirmishes. Excellent hunters—when they go out to kill a deer, you may be sure of their succeeding."[1]

The Delaware hunters going west in search of buffalo soon found themselves fighting the Pawnee, who also claimed the western part of the Delaware reservation. The outnumbered Delawares stood fast and fought back heroically, winning victory and the respect of their foes. At the 1833 peace conference with the Pawnee, Washington Irving's nephew John Treat Irving described the entrance of the proud Delaware warriors, "glittering with trinkets; their silver ornaments glistening in the sunshine, and their gay ribands fluttering in the wind," a gaudy exterior that did not conceal "that indomitable courage, and thirst for glory, which not even intemperance, and their intercourse with the whites could destroy." They were led by the Delaware war chief Captain Suwannock, who "was without ornament, except a heavy silver plate, resting against his calico hunting-shirt. He was not tall, but muscular, and his eye was as searching as an eagle's. There was a proud curl about his lip; and withal, an iron firmness marked his whole deportment. He seemed to think that the whole weight of anger of the Pawnee nation was about to descend upon himself, and he was ready to meet it."[2]

Courageous, capable, and bold, the Delawares were equal to the challenge of life on the frontier. As the years went by, they became famous throughout the West as traders, trappers, and guides. Wagon trains bound for the West would start from Independence, Missouri, just east of the Delaware reservation, and would hire Delaware guides and hunters to help them find their way. Many travelers along the Oregon Trail, the Santa Fe Trail, and other trails west owed their lives to the guidance the Delawares gave them.

The Delawares Make Their Mark

Elsewhere in the West, the Delawares made their mark. They traveled far and wide as trappers and traders, from Canada to Mexico to the Pacific Coast. John James Audubon traveled extensively with the distinguished Delaware scout Black Beaver, exploring the wildlife of the continent. The famed explorer and first Republican nominee for President, John C. Fremont, also used Delaware scouts on his exploration trips. The largest expedition, in 1845, had twelve Delaware scouts, including Chief Anderson's grandson James Secondine, who saved the life of the famed frontiersman Kit Carson. In 1846, when the exploring party reached California, the Mexican-American War broke out, and the expedition suddenly turned into a military mission. The Delawares, with what Fremont called "remarkable courage and fidelity,"[3] ended up guiding the force that captured California for the Union.

To the South, in East Texas, the Absentee Delawares were becoming influential. They maintained good relations with the Mexicans and later the Texans, and time and again acted as go-betweens to the hostile tribes of the Plains such as the Comanches. The Delaware trader Jim Shaw was a good friend of Sam Houston; he and other Delawares helped save the lives of the Texan negotiators after a massacre of Comanche chiefs. On another occasion, the Delaware guide and interpreter Jack Harry saved the lives of Comanches from a murderous band of Texan soldiers. These services helped the Absentee Delawares maintain rights to their land and to their profits from trading. In 1853, a formal reservation was established for them in Texas west of Fort Worth, along the Brazos River.

After the death of Chief Anderson, Captain Ketchum, the brother of Anderson's co-chief, Lapinihile, became the principal chief. His name came from an incident in his youth when he had run down a deer on foot. Upon the death of Ketchum in 1857, John Conner was picked to become chief. Conner, a grandson of Chief Anderson, was a formidable man of many accomplishments. Fluent in several languages, he had traveled throughout all parts of the West. His friend the United States Army officer Colonel Richard Irving Dodge said Conner "was justly renowned as having a more minute and extensive personal knowledge of the North American Continent than any other man ever had or probably ever will have."[4] When Conner was chosen as chief, he was living among the Absentee Delawares in Texas, where he owned a large ranch that he left behind to come north to Kansas.

By this time, there was trouble throughout the frontier. Conflict spread after passage of the Kansas-Nebraska Act in 1853 had allowed settlers onto the Delaware reservation, where they stole homes and property with impunity. The railroads laid tracks across the reservation either by means of fraudulent treaties concocted through bribes and alcohol, or simply without any permission at all. To make matters worse, slavery was spreading into Kansas, embroiling the Delawares in a bitter conflict. The territory soon became known as "Bleeding Kansas" because of the continual bloodshed between pro- and anti-slavery factions. The Delawares had always been horrified by slavery, and had always done their best to provide protection for runaway slaves.

In Texas, a new government hostile to all Native Americans, friendly or not, came into power, and in 1859 passed a law expelling all Native

Americans from Texas. The Absentee Delawares and their friends were forced to move north, across the Red River into Oklahoma, which was then known as Indian Territory. Eventually the Absentee Delawares settled near Anadarko in western Oklahoma, as part of the Caddo nation, or lived among the Plains tribes such as the Kiowa and Comanche.

When the Civil War broke out in 1861, the Delawares supported the Union; a year later, 85 percent of the eligible Delaware men in Kansas had volunteered for the Union Army, where they mostly served in special companies of Delaware scouts. But loyal service could not save their homes. After the war, the pressure for their land continued. Their protests against theft by settlers and fraud by the railroads fell on deaf ears. It was time to leave.

Turning to Old Friends

In 1866, the Delawares sold their remaining lands for $2.50 an acre and set out for the south, to lands in Indian Territory they had purchased from the Cherokees. The Cherokees had long been allies and friends of the Delawares. Though the Cherokees were from the Iroquoian language group, and so were not from the Lenape family, both the Cherokees and the Delawares originally shared a similar Eastern Woodlands Indian way of life and a matrilineal political structure. Both had endured a long, stubborn retreat in the face of white settlers, and both eventually turned their faces westward to look for a new life beyond the Mississippi.

In the West, the Cherokees and Delawares, as leaders of the Eastern immigrant tribes, fought side by side against the Osage, and groups of both won their own territories in East Texas. After almost all of the Cherokee nation had been uprooted and forced westward in the Trail of Tears, the Cherokee survivors established themselves in the eastern part of Oklahoma, "Home of the Red Man," which was then simply known as Indian Territory. By the time the Kansas Delawares asked to join them, the Cherokees, like the Delawares, were becoming farmers and ranchers, familiar with the language and customs of the prevailing American culture.

The Cherokees offered land to the Kansas Delawares for a low price, but they also demanded that the Delawares give up their separate identity and become part of the Cherokee nation, entitled to equal rights and protections. The Kansas Delawares reluctantly agreed, thereby ending their identity as Delawares to merge with the more numerous Cherokees, who at this time had a population of around 14,000. A total of 985 Delaware men, women, and children were recorded on the official list of people eligible for lands and a share of the Cherokee national fund; they

Border design.
This decorative Delaware border design is based on one recorded by Frank Speck.

were known thereafter as the Registered Delawares. These Delawares found homes around the Caney River in the northeastern corner of Indian Territory, and slowly re-established themselves once more.

The last of the Delawares had reached the end of the road. After the epic migration eastward recorded in the Red Record and the long retreat westward caused by the European invasion and its aftermath, both the Absentee and the Registered Delaware divisions had come to the end of their travels in Oklahoma, and there they found a home.

Because the Registered Delawares were centered around the town of Bartlesville, these Delawares living in the Cherokee nation also became known as the Bartlesville Delawares. There were many traditionalists among them who were proud to maintain their own identities and customs as Delawares and disliked the fact that technically they were supposed to be Cherokees. There were also many Delaware modernists, such as the influential Journeycake family, who adopted white ways and abandoned the old religion.

When Chief John Conner died, a dispute between the two groups arose over his successor. An assistant chief of Conner's, Charles Journeycake, who like Conner was from the Turtle group, assumed the chieftainship; he was to be the last chief from the government that had been known as the Delaware nation. However, he was also a Christian minister who lived like a white man. The traditionalists refused to recognize him as a head chief, preferring such leaders as Colonel Jackson. The last of the traditionalist leaders, Charles Elkhair of the Turkey group, died in 1935.

In addition to internal disputes, there was friction with the Cherokees. Resentments remained from the Civil War because the Cherokees had fought for the Confederacy while the Delawares had fought for the Union. The Delawares also complained that they were expected to share their national funds with the Cherokees, yet the Cherokees did not share their funds with the Delawares. The Delawares felt that they were not being given fair treatment by the Cherokees and could not win justice in Cherokee courts, so they decided instead to appeal to the federal courts.

Charles Journeycake brought suit on behalf of the Delawares to win money owed them by the Cherokees and money owed them by the United States government for Delaware property in Kansas. In 1894, the case was argued before the United States Supreme Court. The Delawares won. But their satisfaction was short-lived. Other disputes arose over mineral rights; even over the question of who owned the land that the Delawares had bought and paid for. The Delawares had to file suit against the Cherokees once again in 1898. The educated Delaware modernists Richard C. Adams and George Bullette represented the Delawares in this long, frustrating lawsuit, which slowly worked its way up to the Supreme Court. During the years of struggle and delay in Washington, D.C.,

Adams worked to gain sympathy for the Delaware cause by lobbying Congress and by publishing several illustrated books and pamphlets on Delaware history and previously unrecorded Delaware traditions.

Meanwhile, Oklahoma, as it was now called, was overrun by white settlers. The United States policy became focused on forced assimilation of the remaining Native Americans by the "allotment" policy. Communally owned tribal lands were cut up into fixed allotments for each tribal member, and tribal governments were then dissolved. The effect was to scatter the Native Americans onto individual plots, each like a frail lifeboat on an increasingly stormy sea.

Finally, in 1904, the Supreme Court handed down its decision. Adams and the Delawares had lost. The court ruled that the Cherokees had not had the right to sell the Delawares the land in the first place, because the Cherokees couldn't own any land either. The United States' position was that no Indian, as an Indian, could ever own land; final rights always belonged to the United States, which could, at most, grant occupancy to the Indian. However, an Indian who gave up tribal citizenship and became a United States citizen could own land—provided he or she could pay the taxes.

By this time, the Cherokee Nation was being abolished, with the land broken up into individual allotments. The 200 surviving Registered Delawares were entitled to individual plots of about 160 acres each, which were allotted to them. Although many plots were sold to white people, some Delawares managed to hang on to a few scattered plots, even through the ecological disaster of the 1930s Dust Bowl, and pass at least some portion on to their descendants. These fragments are all that is left today of the land of the Delawares.

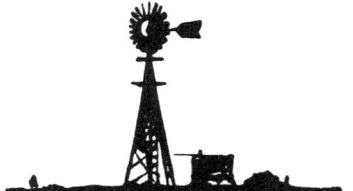

Windmill.
The windmill is a symbol of the Great Plains with its restless winds.

Strangers in Their Own Land

The intention of the allotments had been to assimilate the Native Americans by making them live like white people. Native Americans were made United States citizens, which gave them the right to own land but also subjected them to taxes and various laws, such as those governing property rights and education, that could be at odds with tribal customs and beliefs. The Delawares, and Native Americans everywhere, were being told to disappear. They were treated as strangers in their own land. In response, as the nineteenth century ended and the twentieth century began, a pan-Indian consciousness arose. The tribes by this time had begun mixing and intermarrying, so narrow tribal identities became less important than the fact of being an Indian. The tribes helped each other hold on to essential parts of Indian consciousness in the face of the prevailing American culture.

An important part of this movement became the Native American Church, whose sacrament is peyote (a psychoactive substance contained in a wild cactus). In the 1880s, the use of peyote was adopted by the Absentee Delawares of western Oklahoma from their Kiowa and Comanche friends, who had received it from Mexican tribes familiar with peyote since aboriginal times. Taken as part of religious ceremony, it produces vivid visions and profound emotions that are believed to help clear the heart and bring one closer to harmony with the world of the spirits. The context and control embodied in the ceremony are all-important to guiding the peyote experience for the benefit of the participants.

In the final days of the frontier, the Indian survivors turned inward to hold on to their way of life, and a Delaware-Caddo man named John Wilson became one of the most influential religious leaders of the early Native American Church. Wilson developed the Big Moon Rite, named after the shape of the altar inside the sacred tipi. This rite incorporates Christian elements along with the Native American elements such as the vision quest, pipe, water drum, rattle, and fan. A variant with less Christian influence, the Little Moon Rite later became the most common form of worship. Despite continued government harassment, the Native American Church has survived to this day as an important part of Native American culture, especially among the tribes of the Great Plains.

By the time the Native American Church came into being, the Delawares' status as a separate tribe had been abolished in the eyes of the government, but the Delawares of both eastern and western Oklahoma still retained their identity. The Delawares had endured centuries of frustration in being pushed out of their homes. They had suffered many injustices, both intentional and unintentional, at the hands of the United States government. One of the most telling of the government's acts was the establishment in 1946 of the Indian Claims Commission to settle outstanding claims against the United States. After the commission made a settlement, all responsibilities of the United States toward the tribe in question would be terminated. The tribe would be considered dissolved, extinct, and would be expected to disappear. This policy was known as "termination."

Despite the harsh intention of the law, Native American tribes, including the Delawares, filed suit, seeking what monetary justice they could find. A group of eastern emigrant tribes, including the Stockbridge-Munsies of Wisconsin that were recognized as a separate Delaware group by the government, won a $1.3 million settlement. The 6,446 descendants of the Registered Delawares and the 1,480 members of the Absentee Delawares, known as the Delaware Tribe of Western Oklahoma, also brought suit. They wanted to receive compensation for unfairly low land prices they had been forced to accept when they left their lands in Indiana

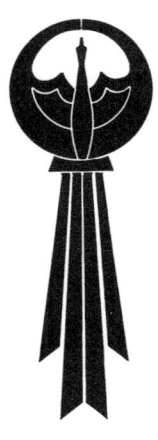

Waterbird.
The waterbird, here drawn from a jewlery design, is a symbol associated with the Native American Church.

and Kansas, and they won more than $15 million in settlements. To date, distribution of the funds among the Registered Delawares has been held up by unresolved disputes with the Cherokees and disagreement over the use of the funds.[5] The Western Delawares have received their portion, and have used their share to support tribal health, housing and administrative programs, and to open a Western Delaware Tribal Museum in Anadarko, which includes among its exhibits a replica set of the Red Record tablets, depicted on page 49.

Today, the more than 13,000 descendants of the Delawares can be found throughout America. They are generally well-educated and prosperous; many can be found in the largest cities, in positions of influence. Small communities of descendants can be found in Kansas, Wisconsin, and New York, as well as in Canada and Oklahoma. An important traditional leader among the Oklahoma Delawares of Bartlesville was Nora Thompson Dean, who died in 1984, and who preserved the Delaware language and customs so they might be appreciated by a new generation. New Jersey descendants known as the Sand Hill Indians, although unrecognized by the government, maintain many Native American traditions and have recently managed to recreate a Delaware village near to New York City. And in August of 1992, a new tribal body dedicated to preserving Delaware culture was born with the formation of The Delaware Nation Grand Council of North America, representing all of the major Delaware groups of Canada and the United States. Its headquarters are in Ohio, near where the Delawares lived on the eve of the Revolutionary War, in what the Red Record calls the Talega Country.

A Retrospective

The Delawares have had an impact on American history out of proportion to their numbers. Before the European invasion, they were influential as the core group of the largest Native American language group in North America, the Lenape family. This influence persisted, despite their heavy losses, even after the European invasion.

The border zone between the expanding white world and the shrinking native world was always present in American consciousness as "The Frontier." Throughout the history of the American frontier, from the 1620s to the 1890s, the Delawares played an important role. They established relations with all of the colonial powers who came to this continent, and, with William Penn, set the standard for successful white-Indian relations. One of the Delaware chiefs at this time, Tamanend, was such an example of virtue that he was later adopted as "St. Tammany, the Patron Saint of America."

Even after they were forced out of their Delaware River lands in the early 1700s, the Delawares re-established themselves in Pennsylvania—where, in peaceful, hard-working communities, they demonstrated how they could be good neighbors to the whites—and in Ohio—where they gathered their eastern relatives and friends together, prepared to defend their rights should the hand of friendship be refused. When the Delawares were rebuffed by the English after war broke out between England and France, a formidable series of attacks by the Delawares of the East and the West showed they were not to be trifled with.

When the American Revolution broke out, it was Delaware diplomats in 1776 that kept the peace on the frontier, enabling the United States to get on its feet. After the Revolution was over, Delaware warriors repaid broken American promises by helping to crush the American armies coming into the Midwest. Every battle depleted the Delawares' numbers, but when they spoke, the tribes of the frontier listened. Their refusal to join with Tecumseh helped doom his cause. But when by 1820 they could no longer see a future in the East, they turned instead to the West, leading the movement of the Eastern tribes to find new homes beyond the Mississippi. Established at last in Texas and Kansas, they were a crucial part of the formative years of each state, and guided travelers, settlers, and explorers as far as the Pacific Coast. At the same time, as traders, they were among the first to acquaint the free tribes of the West with the white invasion that was approaching them, and helped save their tribal friends from some of the invasion's worst effects. Their home bases in Kansas and Texas were eventually taken from them, and they were driven to Oklahoma, where the end of the frontier found them in 1890.

Reduced to a few remnants, the Delawares continued to speak out for their rights before Congress and the Supreme Court. Even as they blended into the mainstream culture, they worked to keep their traditions alive through their ancient rituals, the Native American Church, and the modern Pan-Indian movement, which has helped spark the revival of ecological awareness. Today, as citizens of the United States and Canada, the descendants of the Delawares enrich white culture with their Native American roots, as they continue to seek a blend of the best of both worlds.

Perhaps the greatest impact that the Delaware Indians have had on American history has yet to be fully realized. They left us a legacy—the Wallam Olum or Red Record—which has much to teach us, if we can learn to read it. As a product of the historical tradition that preceded ours, the Red Record offers a new starting point for American history, and for our national identity.

Chapter Seven

Out of the Shadows

The cultural identity of a nation is rooted as much in legend as it is in history. Most of the people of the world look back with wonder and pride to a body of tales that defines their sense of who they are and where they came from. Like the Red Record, these tales begin with myths, grand descriptions of the sacred powers and patterns that underlie the world. Gradually, as events proceed, the tales shift their focus from the divine to the human world, ending with accounts of specific people and incidents that can generally be accepted as historical facts.

Any similarities between the Red Record and other tales of creation, flood, and a search for a homeland are not evidence of any direct influence, but instead show how similar stories have arisen among different cultures as answers to the mysteries of nature and human existence. The Old Testament of the Bible, for instance, tells of the origins of the Hebrew tribes of Palestine thousands of years ago. Its earliest sections, Genesis and Exodus, contain, as does the Red Record, accounts of the Creation of the world and a great Flood, as well as descriptions of the emergence of the Hebrew nation and the migration to a promised land. The miraculous crossing of the Red Sea in Exodus parallels the Red

Record's account of the miraculous crossing of the Bering Strait on the ice.

Another set of stories is told in Greek myths. The creation myth in Hesiod's *Theogony* echoes many of the elements to be found in the earliest sections of the Red Record. Hesiod describes how first there was swirling chaos, then the Earth and the abyss came into being, as well as Eros. From chaos came night and Erebus; from them came day, while from the Earth came heaven, the Titans, and the gods, with Zeus winning the final victory over the forces of disorder.

In addition to such creation myths, other Greek tales go on to mix descriptions of real places, such as Athens and Crete, and possibly real people, such as Minos, with apparently symbolic characters, such as Theseus and the Minotaur. When historical facts are presented as part of such a mix, their real significance can be missed. Chroniclers of genius such as Homer described life and war as far back as the Bronze Age, but scholars dismissed the *Iliad* as having no basis in fact until Heinrich Schliemann, at the end of the nineteenth century, proved them wrong by unearthing Troy and Mycenae. Recent excavations at Thera are proving that there may even be some truth in Plato's careful descriptions of Atlantis.

Like the Greeks, the Romans had their own poetic-historical tradition of their origins, the *Aeneid* by Virgil. It tells of the adventures of Aeneas, who, after the fall of Troy, led the Trojan refugees in a search for a new homeland, a quest that led eventually to Italy, where their descendants would found the city of Rome. Knowledge of such ancient and glorious ancestors was a basis for pride in being a Roman during the days of the Roman Empire.

In other countries, other national traditions supplied a foundation for their cultures. The Norse sagas, like the Red Record, included creation myths along with a chronicle of several generations of heroes, many of them historical figures like Eric the Red and Leif Ericson. In India, the earliest days are chronicled in the *Rig-Veda*, which describes how Aryans first migrated into India thousands of years ago; the *Ramayana* and the *Mahabharata* are other multi-generationsl epics that describe the origins of the nations that are the direct ancestors of those in India today. In China, there are ancient chronicles such as the *Shih Chi* describing the origins of what would later become China. These and other tales begin with the mythical period of the Yellow Emperor and the shadowy Xia Dynasty. As the tales progress into the Shang Dynasty and beyond, they become increasingly grounded in historical fact.

In Africa, which did not have the written traditions found in these other regions, history was kept by professionals trained to exactly preserve facts through memory. The griots, the oral historians of West Africa, have

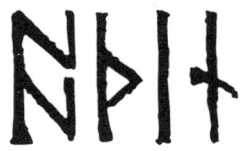

Runes.
The ancient Germanic alphabet called runes was especially adapted to carving in wood.

Bantu symbol.
Among Bantu people, this symbol meant "future days."

proven many times their ability to remember facts over many generations, as exactly as if the facts had been written down on paper. It was a griot, for example, who provided the details about Alex Haley's lost African past in *Roots*. In South Africa, the vivid and suspenseful tales of the Bantu were preserved only in oral form, until Vasamazulu Credo Mutwa wrote them down in 1966 in *Indaba, My Children*. These stories also begin in the earliest days with tales of creation and go on to describe ancient wars and heroes and a great migration of the tribes southward into South Africa. The tales end with the coming of the Portugese in the sixteenth century. In the course of these stories, incidents are described that at first seem incredible—the account of the rise and fall of an ancient Phoenican slave empire in southern Africa was at first thought to be a myth but has since been confirmed by archaeology.

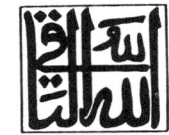

Arabic words.
"Allah the Eternal" reads this Arabic inscription.

Recent archeology has also confirmed the descriptions in the Koran, the sacred text of Islam, and in Islamic legends of the wealthy lost city of Ubar, which was said to have been suddenly destroyed by God because of its wickedness. Using evidence from satellite photography, archeologists in 1992 located what Lawrence of Arabia once called "the Atlantis of the sands" within the part of Oman known as the Empty Quarter. There they discovered that Ubar had indeed been suddenly destroyed when a cavern beneath it caved in, and much of the city vanished into the abyss.[1]

In South America, the history of the Inca Empire and its predecessors can be reconstructed through archeology and from the legends of the native culture that still endures. Although writing was not used in ancient South America, there was a well-developed oral tradition. Among the Incas there was a special class, the *amautas*, among the wisest and most honored, who were responsible for preserving the historical traditons. According to the Spanish chronicler Pedro de Cieza de Léon, writing shortly after the conquest of the Incas, these oral historians were motivated by a desire "that the people might be animated by the recital of what had passed in other times." The artfully composed "romances" of former days were handed down and taught with care. The Spanish chronicler says, "By this plan from the mouths of one generation the succeeding one was taught, and they can relate what took place five hundred years ago as if only ten years had passed."[2]

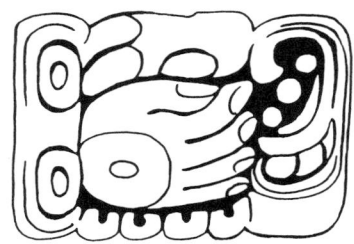

Mayan glyph.
This Mayan glyph comes from a temple at Palenque, Guatemala.

In Central America and Mexico, spectacular monuments were carved and constructed by the Olmecs as early as 1,000 B.C. but written records were lacking until the Maya consolidated their city-states more than a thousand years later. In addition to a writing system, the Maya also perfected an advanced calender and left precise dates. The Maya records include the Hieroglyphic Stairway in the Maya city of Copan, the longest carved inscription in pre-Columbian America. Its more than 1,200 glyphs relate a mythological and dynastic chronology, like the Red Record, telling of the origins and history of Copan up to the moment when the inscription was dedicated in the year 755. The Maya also wrote many books, although only three postclassic Maya books are known to have survived. The Mayan genesis, the *Popul Vuh* (Book of Counsel) was recorded in 1802 by a parish priest who was allowed to copy an even earlier copy made by a Quiché Maya Indian around 250 years before.[3] Like the Red Record, the *Popul Vuh* exists now only in the form of this most recent manuscript copy; the first copy and the original manuscript have been lost.

The Mexica, better known as the Aztecs, also kept many written records, some of which, such as the *Mendoza Codex* and *Telleriano-Remiensis Codex*, escaped the wanton destruction of the Spanish conquerors. These records and other native traditions describe the ancient migration of the Aztecs from out of the north into the valley of Mexico. These traditions are not dismissed as legends, but are accepted as a fundamental part of Mexican history. One incident in the journey, the vision of the eagle seizing the snake—the vision that led to the founding of Mexico City in 1325—is proudly featured in the center of the Mexican flag.

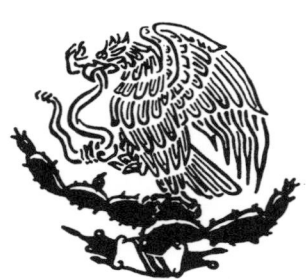

Mexican flag. The national emblem of Mexico, from the Mexican flag, refers back to Aztec legends.

A Lack of Chronicles of Ancient North America

North of the Rio Grande, there is no history that matches the scope and completeness of the Red Record. Like the great historical narratives found elsewhere in the world, the Red Record spans the gap from mythological to historical times. It begins with creation myths common to many cultures—myths of primordial lands rising from the waters, a great Flood, and the victory of a great hero over a devouring serpent—and ends with events that appear in other historical records, including the coming of European explorers and colonists.

It is also remarkable in that although it is brief, it includes so many of the essential elements of what is commonly defined as a historical record. The obviously mythological sections are clearly marked as Books I and Book II. Book III is transitional, and may include elements of legend as well as history. But the main part of the Red Record, Books IV and V, which forms the most obviously historical narrative, has a clear chronological scale in the succession of the ninety-six chiefs, and an account of a journey that is remarkably systematic and accurate. The style in this main section consists entirely of plain statements of fact, with none of the divine interventions characteristic of myths and legends.

The Red Record is the United States' only parallel to the ancient tales of the rest of the world. But why in the United States are there no other chronicles of the ancient past? There were many forms of historical records among the Native American tribes, but these have either not survived, not been interpreted, or not been revealed to the uninitiated.

The destruction of Native American cultures is the main reason we do not have more records of ancient times. The Natchez in Mississippi, for instance, had written archives recording a tradition that went back through forty-five to fifty successive chiefs, but these archives were burned by the French in 1734 when, in response to a revolt, they destroyed the Natchez nation.[4] The English-speaking colonists were especially ruthless in excluding the Native Americans and their cultures from the new nation that became the United States. Native Americans were not welcome because their presence was seen as a denial of the colonists' right to take possession of the continent. The colonists had to see the land as empty, so they erased the people and history that were already there.

Another reason the United States has no ancient history besides the Red Record is the difficulty of confirming and interpreting other surviving native historical records. As products of a non-Western tradition, they are not amenable to Western standards of proof. The usual archeological evidence of "bones and stones" does not apply; the names of past heroes cannot be read from skeletons and tools. There are no written records from those times that can give corroborative proof, such as the Egyptian hieroglyphic records of Biblical events. Many inscriptions, decorations, and petroglyphs (rock carvings or drawings) have been found across the continent, but these records are all symbolic and mnemonic in nature. The ancient people who created them assumed that living memory would preserve their meaning; although individuals might die and generations pass away, their culture would live on. They could not have imagined the holocaust that would engulf them, a destruction so total that even memory became extinct.

Chumash sun. The Chumash, a Southern California tribe, used this petroglyph to represent the sun.

A third reason for the lack of ancient history is the reluctance of native people to reveal their traditions to the uninitiated. Outsiders have so often scorned, misunderstood, and distorted what they have learned that traditional elders quite understandably want to keep their knowledge to themselves. Among Native American cultures that have survived relatively intact, such as the Hopi of Arizona, there is a body of knowledge, records, and traditions reaching far back into the past, as well as into the future—secret lore, including some carved into tablets, that will probably never be revealed.

In discussing this tendency of the Native Americans to be secretive about intimate aspects of their culture, Ojibwa Chief George Copway says, "This secrecy is not generally known by those people who have searched with interest the Indian, and traced him in all his wanderings to get an idea of his religion and his worship, which however absurd they may have seemed, have nevertheless been held in so rigid respect that he has formed for it a cloak of almost impenetrable mystery."[5] This cloak of mystery has undoubtedly preserved many traditions from the persecutions of well-meaning but misguided lawmakers. In fact, it was not until 1979, with the passage of the Native American Religious Freedom Act, that Native Americans began to be allowed to practice their ancient religion without fear of interference.

Considering what has happened to the Delaware nation, it is surprising that the Red Record was ever revealed to white people. The disasters that befell the Delawares after the Europeans came shattered their national family and scattered them far from their homeland. Their customs were ridiculed, their beliefs were denied, and they were dismissed as savages. Missionaries converted great numbers to Christian teachings and made them deny their culture. So it is little wonder that long ago, Delaware traditionalists became very reluctant to tell white people about their most intimate beliefs. They remained proud of who they were and did all they could to safeguard the heritage of what they considered a better way of life.

It is not then surprising that we can find no mention of the Red Record in the writings of missionaries and other white visitors. Yet William Penn may have overheard a chant much like it in the late 1600s. As Penn's friend John Oldmixon reported it, "While the Captain General was in the Bagnio [sweat lodge], he first sang all the Acts of the Nation he was of . . . then those of his Ancestors, who were Nobles and Generals in the Country; and last of all, his own."[6] As late as the late 1800s, a long mythological and historical chant was still being recited each year among the Shawnees on the Quapaw Reservation in Oklahoma, which was then still Indian Territory. Daniel G. Brinton tried to obtain a copy of the chant and was rebuffed, for "They say that to repeat it to a white man would bring disasters to their nation."[7] When, in 1820, the Red Record was presented by the Delawares to a white man (see page 5), Americans were given an opportunity to learn about the earliest days, when North America was entirely in the stewardship of the Native Americans. Almost two centuries have passed, and still the Red Record has not had the attention it so richly deserves.

In the past, contemptuous dismissal left too many native traditions unrecorded even if they were revealed. The blind piety that drove the earliest explorers, conquerors, and colonists would not admit the truth of any other historical traditon except that recorded in the Bible. Other existing traditions were ignored as worthless or condemned as works of the Devil. The attitude of one Spanish priest, Father José de Acosta, was typical, "It is no matter of any great importance to know what the Indians themselves report of their beginning, being more like unto dreams than to true histories."[8] Another Spanish chronicler reported native traditions with distaste, saying, "I will merely mention a few to illustrate the folly and blindness in which they lived."[9] Such attitudes resulted in lost native history throughout the New World.

It is now time to reclaim what was lost, to remember what was forgotten. Native cultures all over the world are now speaking out, trying to teach us again about the secrets of life and the Earth, about the past, and about the future. Native Americans represent a tradition of partnership with this land that is thousands of years old, yet remains the best hope for our own future surival. As the anthropologist John Collier says, they "speak to us from out of our long foregone home, and what hears them is the changeless, eternal part of us imprisoned and immured by our social epoch even as the Indian societies were imprisoned and immured by us in the century behind. Just as our own buried depths predict a world future and belong to it, so these outwearing, ancient Indian societies predict a world future and belong to it."[10]

The Red Record speaks from the time before the imprisonment began; before the prison was even conceived. It is a guiding thread that can lead us back, out of the sad labyrinth of history since Columbus, past the mistakes and regrets, past the accidents and destruction, to rediscover our lost innocence in an age of wonder.

Appendix

Mapping the Migration

It is possible to map a systematic reconstruction of the migration route described in the Red Record. During this reconstruction, we will test the accuracy of the geographical descriptions in the Red Record, for if the account does indeed describe a migration out of Asia and across North America, then it should include not only indications of the most important landmarks, but should also accurately measure the distance between them.

The first step of this test is to plot out the described journey in the Red Record. Figure A-1 is a chart graphing the population movements indicated in the historical narrative of Book III, Book IV, and most of Book V. This chart was made by simply allowing each indication of a direction in the symbol or words of a verse to shift the population one square in that direction. The number of the verse that caused the shift to be made on the graph appears next to the newly established population center. If only one direction indicator appears in a verse, then the shift is only one square. If direction indicators appear in both the symbol and the words of a verse, then the movement is two squares, and the extra amount of movement is shown by an arrow. In certain cases, where the narrative makes it clear

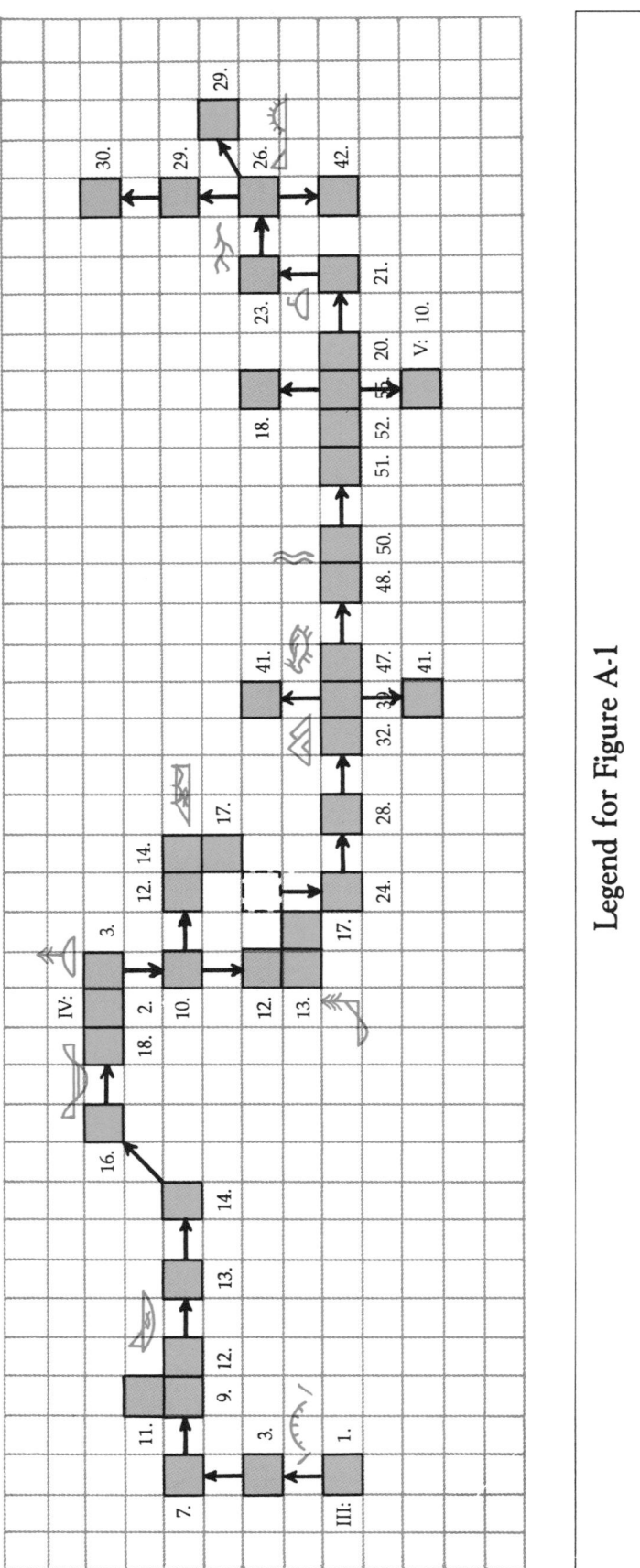

Legend for Figure A-1

	The Mississippi River. (IV:49)
	The Allegheny Mountains. (V:19–20)
	The Susquehanna River. (V:24)
	The Atlantic Ocean shoreline, at dawn. (V:26)

	The forests and shoreline of Akolaki to the south. (IV:13)
	The mountainous hunting and fishing country to the east. (IV:14)
	A mountain range bordering the Great Plains. (IV:29)
	An indication of buffalo herds. (IV:37)

	Indications of storms and cold. (III:2)
	A shoreline with fishing. (III:12)
	Shores on either side of a frozen sea. (III:16–19)
	Evergreen forests in Akomen to the east. (III:20;IV:1;IV:8)

Figure A-1. Lenape symbols for selected landscape features plotted on a graph of the Lenni Lenape's movements. **If a word or a symbol indicates a shift of the population, the population moves one square in the indicated direction. If both the word and symbol indicate direction, the movement is two squares in that direction (arrows show the extra amount of movement). Numbers indicate the book and verse where the information is found.**

that a shift refers to a breakaway group, the main population center is left in place. In addition to indicators of directional movement, there are many details of landscape, wildlife, and climate noted along the way. Some of the symbols for these landscape features have been placed according to the Red Record's account of where they were encountered.

Figure A-1 reveals a migration path that consistently moves east, including a curve first to the north, then to the south. This chart of a long, gradual eastward migration through different landscape features forms a rough map, on which the distance and direction between features can be measured by squares on the grid. The path does not double back or zigzag erratically. This same basic path is found if either the words or the symbols are plotted alone. The only split is explained in Book IV, verses 10–14.

The next step is to test whether or not this rough map corresponds to the actual map of North America. This can best be seen by retracing the journey back in time, from modern times into the distant past. The identification of noted landmarks such as the Allegheny Mountains and the Susquehanna River is clear. We also can identify the symbols for the Mississippi River and the White River in Indiana. From these known points in the East and Midwest, we can test whether the scale of distances between these features is reflected by the map of North America. We find that they do not match; the steps from the Alleghenies to the East Coast are smaller than from the Mississippi to the Alleghenies. But other landscape features are indicated in the Red Record further westward: a great range of mountains like the Rockies and the "Yellow River," which could be the Yellowstone. In addition, herds of buffalo, a well-known feature of the Great Plains, are described. But testing the distances between these features, we again find that when we go farther westward, to points earlier and earlier in the migration, the length of the steps between landscape features increases.

This discrepancy indicates that the most recent stages of the journey have been described in more detail, with smaller increments of movement, while earlier stages have been described in more generalized terms, with larger steps, a characteristic of any story that has been preserved in memory, since people tend to remember recent events more exactly. In fact, we can see this change in length of the steps happening in a gradual curve, as we move back in time to the region of the Rocky Mountains.

In an earlier time, west of the Rockies, the Lenape are described as sustaining themselves by gathering plant foods rather than hunting, after having come south from a much colder region. This reflects the differences between the Great Plateau and the Canadian Rockies. Earlier still in the story, we continue to find correspondences between the landscape features mentioned in the Red Record and the landscape features still to be found on the map today; the "tall pine country, seashore country" (IV:13) matches the region today called the Northwest Coast; the "fishing country, mountain country, game herd country" (IV:14) matches the Yukon and Northwest territories. But we also find a mismatch of distances; the scale of steps seems larger still, and more than one step seems to be missing. However, the explanation can be found in the text, for the Red Record describes this period as a confusing time. The tribe had divided earlier (around 380 A.D. according to a count of the generations), between those who had gone south along the shore and those who had continued east into the hunting country inland. After a period of great trouble, the unity and historical traditions of the Lenape were apparently restored by Olumapi, History Man (IV:23), who is identified as having invented the first written records.

Other landmarks even further to the west enable us to find our bearings and to establish an average scale of distances. First, there is a forest land that matches the Yukon valley, and to the west, a wide ice-covered strait, described in unusual detail, which must be the Bering Strait.

The earliest section of the Lenape journey takes place in Book III. Figure A-1 on page 184 shows a great distance being traveled northeastward during this period, from a starting point deep within Asia to the Bering Strait. The distance and direction indicates that this would have been a trip across eastern Siberia, from a starting point near China. The position of the landscape features noted along the way confirms this; first, there are indications of the cold mountains along the northern Chinese border, then the river plains of the Lena basin, then the barren storm-torn mountains to the northeast, and the maritime environment beside the Bering Sea.

So it seems to be true that the landscape features noted at various points in the journey correspond to real locations. The final test is to see how well this pattern of landmarks, separated by measured distances represented by steps on the grid, corresponds to the actual map.

In the modern era, ships and satellites have explored the contours of the land from the sea and from the air. Native people walking the land, such as the Lenape, had earlier come to know it on a more intimate scale, bit by bit. Only rarely, such as in a document like the Red Record, can the sum of such accumulated firsthand knowledge of the land be compared to the findings of the modern era. For accuracy and fairness in the test, it is important to use the most distortion-free map possible.

Since making any map of the world involves projecting a spherical surface onto a flat sheet, every world map will have some distortion. (The Mercator Projection, for instance, makes Greenland appear huge, as big as South America.) Any distortion prevents the accurate plotting of the steps described in the Red Record onto an actual landscape, and comparison to the features found there. The best map to use, therefore, would be one that has the least average distortion over the route of the Lenape migration, a route that goes from Asia to the East Coast, almost halfway around the world.

Recently, such a map was invented by the genius of Buckminster Fuller. By wrapping the surface of the globe around the twenty-sided regular solid known as the icosahedron, the Fuller Projection eliminates a significant amount of distortion within each land mass, and avoids having to show Asia separated from America. Even more important, the edges of this icosahedron happen to follow the Lenape migration route, maintaining a consistent scale of distances throughout (see figures A-2 and A-3).

An average scale of distance of about 216 statute (standard) miles (347.62 kilometers) per step (box on the chart) leads to a remarkably accurate correspondence for locations throughout Siberia into North America. The steps are shown on the map as circles instead of squares, to make diagonal steps the same length as lateral or vertical steps. As the journey moves across North America toward its conclusion, the scale of distance per step can be seen to gradually diminish, reflecting the tendency of the "narrators" to remember the most recent parts of the journey in more detail (see Figure A-4 on page 193).

Allowing for this diminishing scale, the amount of correspondence between the descriptions in the Red Record and the actual landscape of North America becomes even more remarkable. Only five adjustments— added steps—are needed to produce a nearly perfect match, and each of these missing steps has at least some historical basis in the Red Record.

As Book IV begins, one eastward step must be added between verses 3 and 10, assuming that the distance of roughly 216 miles per step characteristic of Book III remains constant. Although the narrative in verses 4–7 describes a Lenape campaign against the tribes in the interior of Alaska, it does not explicitly mention an eastward direction.

After this, the Lenape split in two in verse 12. One part of the tribe is described as going to the south, along the shore, but because the shore actually tends to the southeast, one step of southern movement and one step of eastern movement need to be added. The other part of the tribe is described as going to the hunting country eastward. To place this part of the tribe well beyond the Rockies, one step eastward needs to be added to the movement. After a long period of trouble and confusion, Olumapi, History Man appears (IV:23); he is credited with the invention of written records. Apparently the two wings of the tribe reunited at this time, as Olumapi helps to re-establish their history and their identity, so a further adjustment is needed to bring the two halves together at a central point.

Almost none of these extra increments would need to be added if the average distance of the steps at the beginning of Book IV were 25 percent

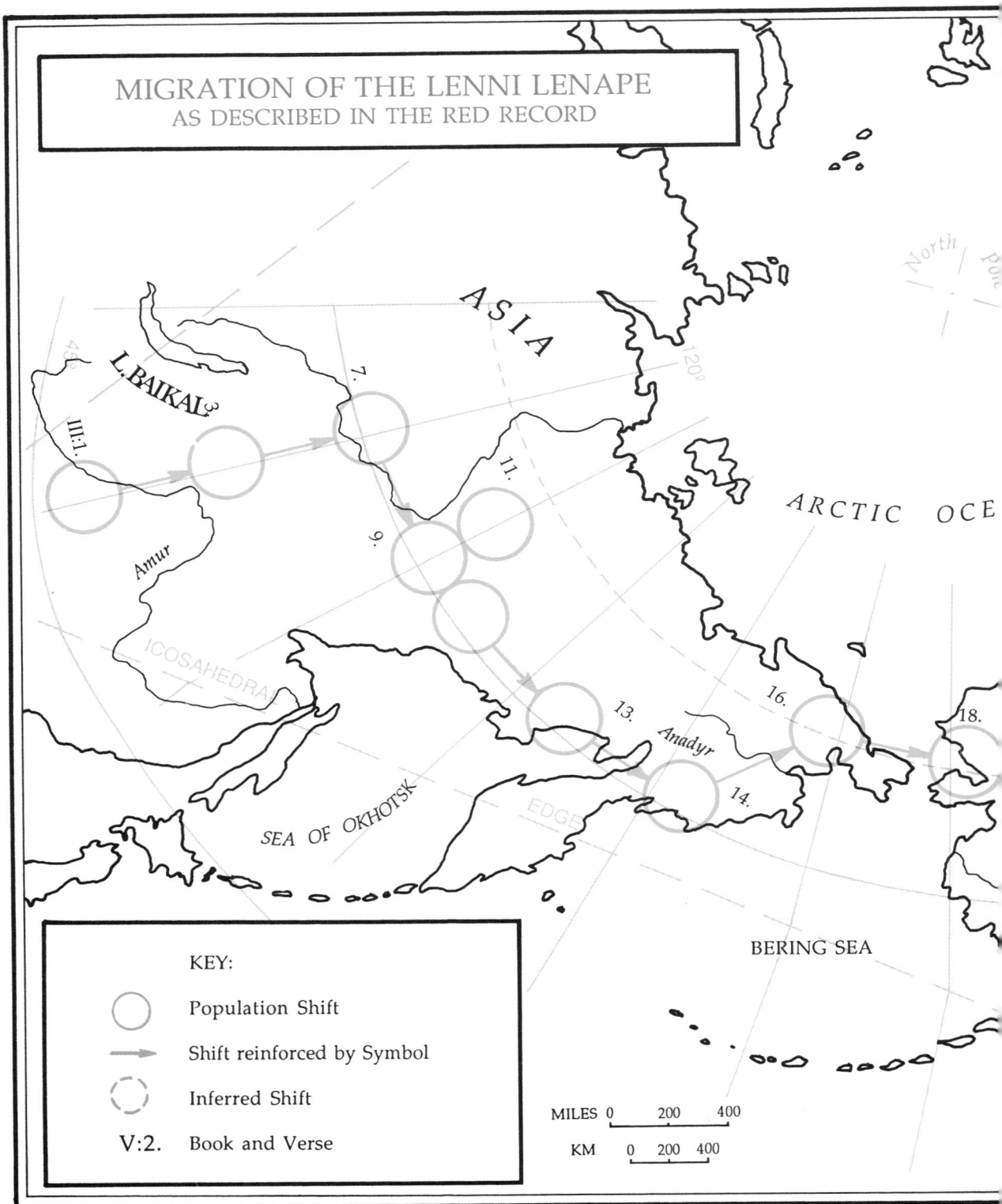

Figure A-2. Migration of the Lenni Lenape as described in the Red Record. The route of the Lenni Lenape from Asia to the North American continent is depicted on a Fuller Projection Map, which has minimal distortion of distances. The book and verse that revealed the movement is noted. Arrows

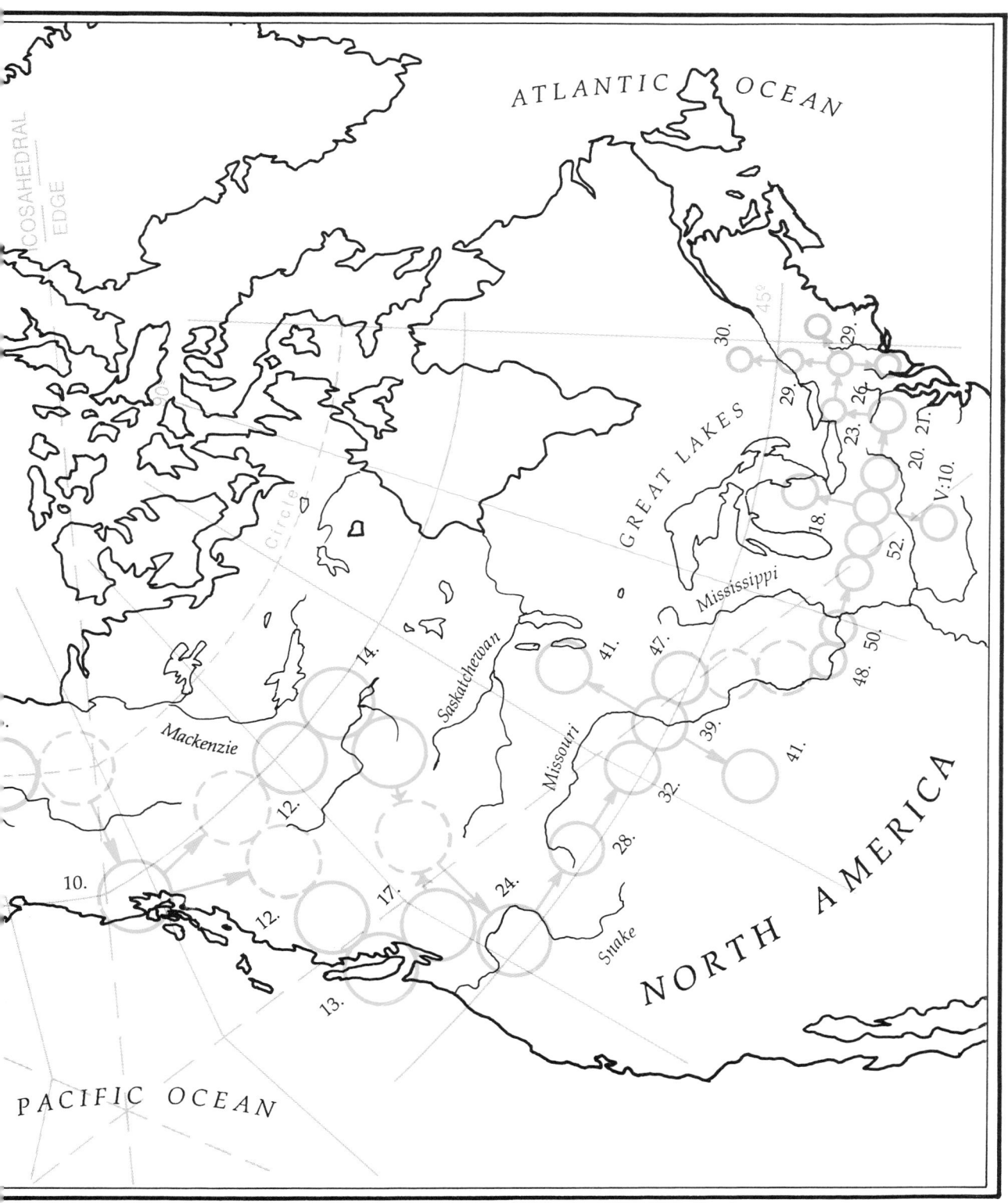

indicate that the movement was described in both the words and symbols. **Solid circles show a new center of population; broken-line circles indicate that the shift has been inferred rather than directly stated in the Red Record.**

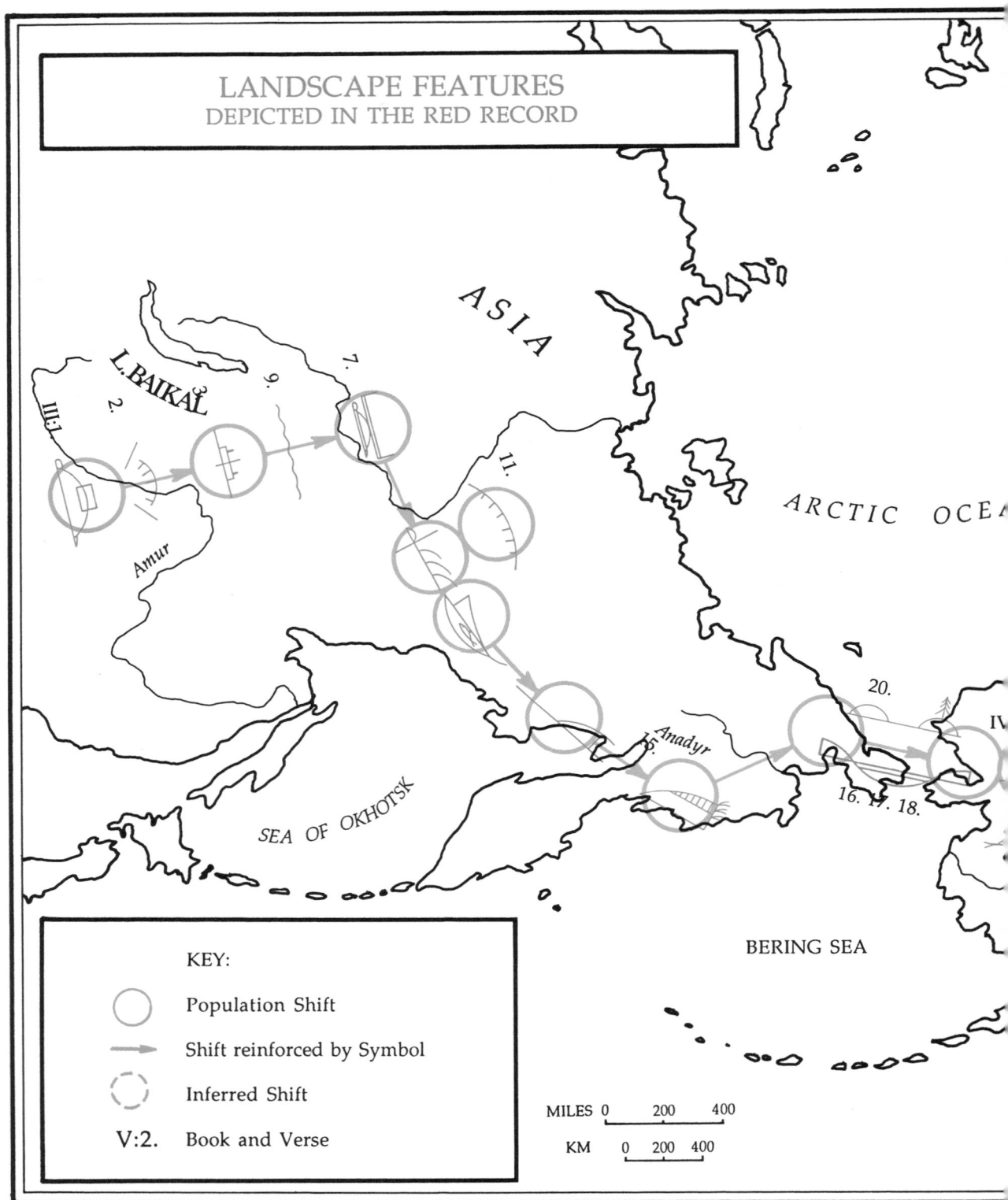

Figure A-3. Landscape features depicted in the Red Record. The migration route of the Lenni Lenape is depicted on a Fuller Projection Map. In addition to information about the steps along the route

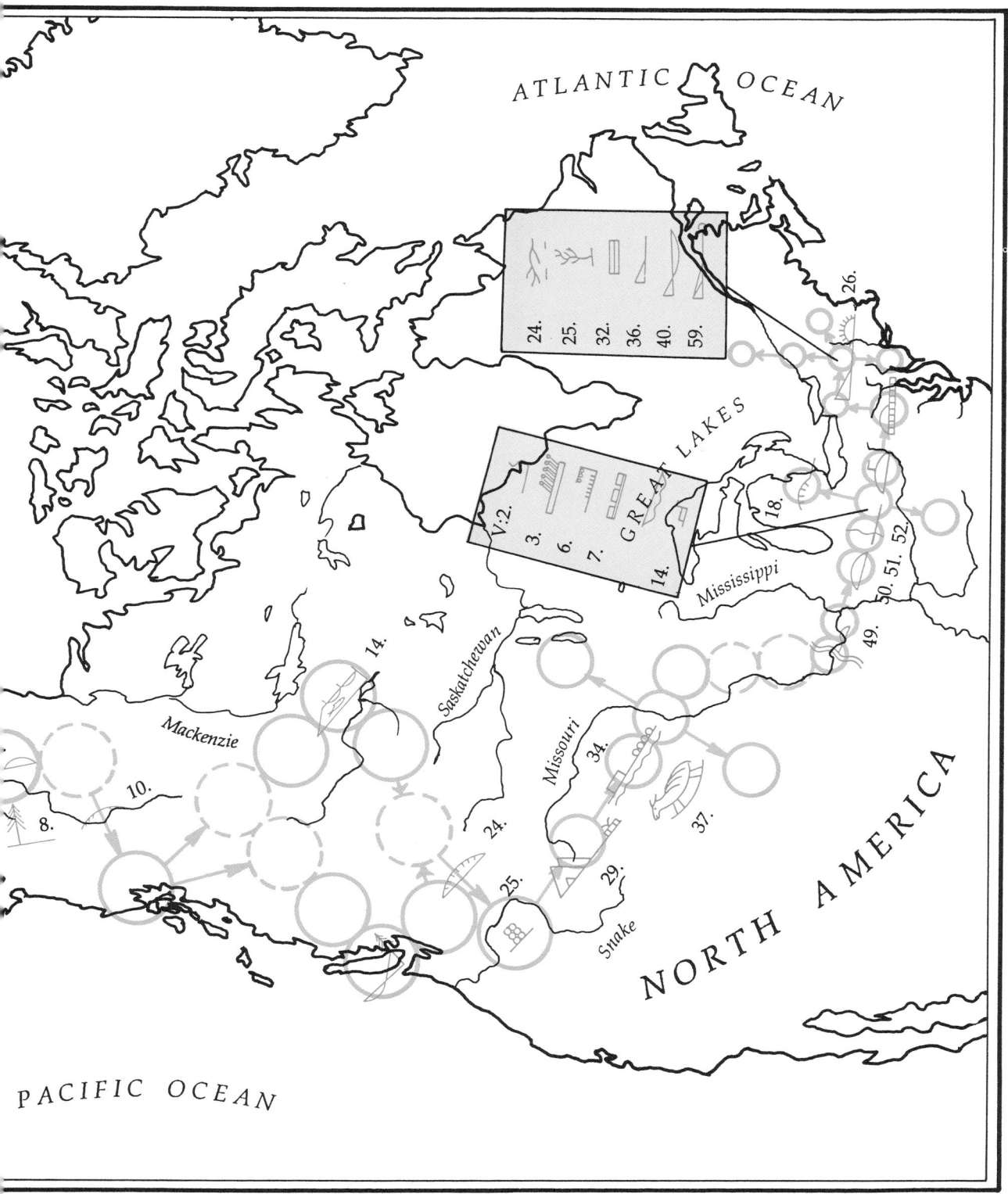

(see Figure A-2), this figure highlights the Lenape symbols for various landscape features the Lenape encountered on their journey. (Legend for the above map appears on next page.)

Legend for Figure A-3

Symbol from Book III:

III:1 A "Turtle Island"; possibly hill country.

III:2 Cold and winds, "icy . . . snowy . . . freezing."

III:3 A plain identified as "the north slope."

III:4 A river linking the "travelers" and the "builders."

III:7 A northern plain, "the turtle land, the great land."

III:9 A hill or "Turtle Island," once the home of the Snakes.

III:11 Indication of cold weather in "the snowy country."

III:12 A seashore with fish in the ocean.

III:13 An eastern land beyond the ocean, "the land of Akomen."

III:15 The eastern land is shown as occupied by Snakes.

III:16–18 Two shorelines with a "frozen sea" between.

III:20 The eastern "evergreen" land and the western "old Turtle Country."

Book IV:

IV:1 The new "evergreen land" in the east.

IV:3 Indications of the forests and the Snakes in "Akomen. . . the good land."

IV:6 The valley of the "Snake hollow."

IV:8 The forests of the "evergreen land."

IV:10 Indication of cold weather.

IV:13 "Akolaki. . . tall pine country, seashore country."

IV:14 "Fishing country, mountain country, game herd country."

IV:24 The cold land in the north left behind by "Frozen One."

IV:25 The crops grown by "Hominy Man."

IV:29 Mountains, and "beyond the pass," the herds of the "Great Plains."

IV:34 The "Yellow River," showing the fruits of the "wide meadows."

IV:35 The "Mighty Bison" of the Great Plains, shown running.

IV:49 The "Mississippi" River, and the land to the east.

IV:50 The Talegas in the east are shown atop a mound.

IV:51 The Talega land, represented as a mound.

IV:52 A river crossed by those "massacred" by "the Talega king."

Book V:

V:2 A river identified as "the Shining Stream."

V:3 "Great crops" are shown growing in the fields.

V:6 "Great harvests" are shown stored safely indoors.

V:7 A land with indications that "the towns were many."

V:8 An indication of "many streams."

V:14 A town in the Talega Country, "along the Ohio."

V:18 Indication of cold in "the northern wastes."

V:19–20 The "Alleghenies" or Talega Mountains.

V:22 To the east, forests in a "rich land" where "it was beautiful."

V:24 A picture of the "Susquehanna" River.

V:25 The trees of "Sassafras Country."

V:26 The Eastern Shore, showing the sun rising from "the Ocean."

V:32 A homeland (triple ground line).

V:36 Again, the trees of the land of "the sassafras."

V:40 A shoreline with the sea to the east (also seen in verses 51, 57, 58, and 60).

V:59 An indication of one or possibly two shorelines, representing the lands of the "north and south."

larger than those in Book III, or approximately 270 miles (434.52 kilometers) instead of 216 miles each. This increase matches the trend that is characteristic of Book IV in which greater distances are related during earlier time periods. But in the interest of consistency and clarity, the steps in Book III and the beginning of Book IV are here kept the same length, and the cause of the mismatch is ascribed to the historical unrest and confusion during this period that made the invention of written records necessary.

Finally, two southeastward steps need to be added between verses 47 and 48, after Opekasit, East Looking (IV:47), initiates a migration to the east. This addition may be needed because this migration would have almost certainly followed the course of the Missouri River, which curves southeastward before it turns to the east to join the Mississippi.

With the addition of these minor adjustments, the painstakingly preserved Stone Age survey of two continents in the Red Record is confirmed by the latest Space Age measurement and display of the landscape.

Distance Per Step

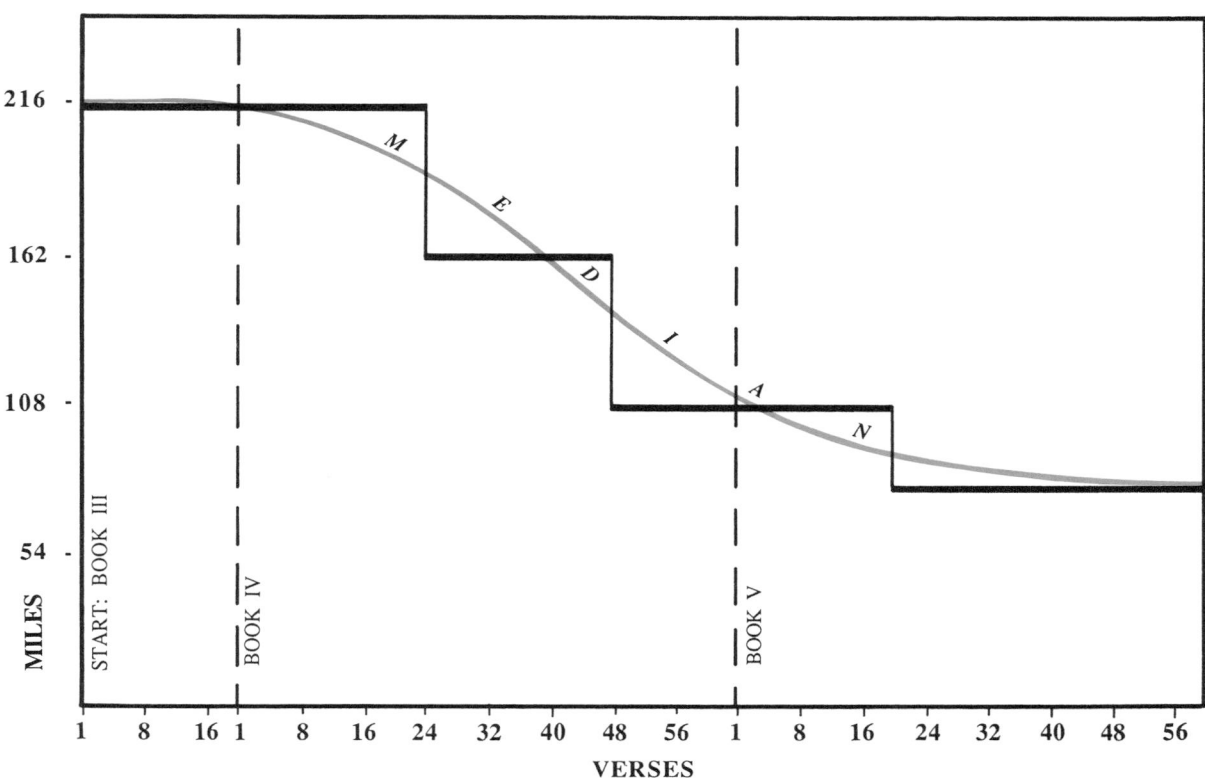

Figure A-4. Distance per step. The graph depicts the decreasing scale of distance in each "step" of the Lenape migration as successive verses move the story toward more recent times.

Translation Notes

The Red Record is difficult to translate not only because many of the original Delaware words survive only in a garbled form, but also because the Delaware language in some cases embraces concepts that have no clear equivalent in English. Some of the choices made in this translation deserve a fuller explanation, not only to show how the English words were determined, but also to show the subtlety and richness of the original Delaware words. Unless otherwise identified, the Delaware words and meanings that do not appear in the Red Record are from Reverend Kampman's excellent dictionary manuscript in the Moravian archives, recording the language as it was spoken in the late eighteenth and early nineteenth centuries, and later annotated by Reverend A.S. Anthony, a Munsee-Delaware, and published by Brinton in 1885 as A *Lenâpé-English Dictionary*.

Essop (I:2–3) is here translated "moved" instead of the more usual "was." The Delaware root *Lissin* means both "to be" and "to do"; since there is no active form of "to be" in English, a more active word was chosen, since action would be needed to bring about the Creation.

Sohalawak (I:4,5,6,14,15; IV:23) was translated as "He causes them" by Rafinesque. Rather than characterize the Great Spirit as male or female, I used the more neutral and active "bringing forth" or "brought forth." Later the word *Sohalawak* is used for Olumapi's invention of written records (IV:23), a creative act of great significance, where it is translated as "began." In all cases, a creative, inventive, generative act is being described.

Owini (I:10,12,16; II:5,8,10) was translated by Rafinesque as "such-they men"; a better definition is "those beings that are," in other words, "life" or "living things."

Nijini (I:18-19; II:2) was translated by Rafinesque as "the Jins" (as in jinn or genies) while others have translated it as "the beings." A better translation that fits the context is "these ancestors." (Compare *Nik* meaning "these, those"; and *Nigani* meaning "the first, foremost.")

Wulamo (II:1; IV:1; V:1), the first word of many of the books of the Red Record, is here translated as long ago." It is an archaic form, which suggests "of yore"; it also has other shades of meaning; compare *Wulamoeii* meaning "truly"; *Wulamoc*, "he speaks truly, true"; *Wulamoewagan*, "truth."

Palliton (II:3,5,7; IV:43-47,53,63; V:15,43) is a general term for warfare, here translated as "destroyed"or "fought." It is usually accompanied by the X-shaped pictograph for war. Kampman's translation of *Palliton*, "to spoil something, to do it wrong," does not take into account the prefix *Palli* meaning "away"; the meaning is closer to "despoil" or "do away with."

Wulaton (III:3; IV:56) has been translated as "to have" and "they won," respectively, to adjust to the different contexts, but in both cases the meaning derives from the prefix *Wulit* meaning "good, right, handsome, pretty, well." Kampman defines *Wulaton* as "to save, to put up"; compare the archaic *Palaton* meaning "to earn, to acquire." *Wullaton Apakchikton* (IV:10) is translated "to grow and/spread there" because of the combination with *Apachtchiechton* meaning "to display, to set something up; to attach one's self to, to fix upon."

Pawasinep Wapasinep (III:13) is here translated as "gloried/in the eastern light," but these two words form a complex rhyme with many intertwined meanings. *Pawa* is a prefix for "dream power" as in *Pawallessin*, "to be rich" (including in dreams). (Compare the Ojibwa word *Pawaanaat* [from Voegelin], meaning "he dreams of him.") Similarly, *Wapa* is a prefix meaning both "white"and "east" (as in the dawn); the Delawares would face the dawn as they prayed, for this was the source of the future, and of spiritual power. (The suffix *–sinep* is a past tense ending.) So the verse suggests that the land to the east, Akomen, was a source of spiritual power, a promised land, a "land of their dreams."

Oligonunk (IV:29) is here translated "beyond the pass"; earlier translators have given "Hollow Mountain over" or "At the place of caves" as suggested by Heckewelder's *Wahlo* (from which is drawn the name of Oley, Pennsylvania) meaning "cave or cavern." Rather than say "hollow mountain," it makes more sense to say "mountain hollow" or "pass."

Wallamolumin (V:5) is translated as "writing the Red Record," reflecting an ongoing process of recording the past. The completed record itself, called the *Wallam Olum* (according to the most-used spelling in the Rafinesque Manuscript) is translated by Rafinesque as "painted and engraved traditions." *Wallam* or *Walam*, from the root *wul–* meaning "pleasurable sensation," is a name for red paint, from the sense "to be fine in appearance, to dress," since a Lenape man painted red was considered to be in "fancy dress." *Olum* seems to come from the root *Ol–* meaning something hollowed, as in an engraved mark. *Olum* is translated by Rafinesque as "tally," referring to the engraved tally sticks traditionally used by the Lenape to keep score in games. Brinton and others therefore translated *Olum* as "score," perhaps also suggesting a musical score, since the symbols served as a mnemonic guide for the performance of a musical chant. But a translation of *Wallam Olum* as "Red Score" overlooks other similar words suggesting antiquity and truthfulness, such as *Wulamoe*, an archaic form meaning "long ago"; *Wulamoeii* "truly"; *Wulamoc* "he speaks truly, true"; and *Wulamoewagan* "truth." To also encompass these meanings suggesting an ancient history or testament, I have therefore translated *Wallam Olum* as "Red Record."

Notes

Part One: Echoes of Ancient Voices

Chapter One

1. Indiana Historical Society, *Walam Olum or Red Score: The Migration Legend of the Delaware Indians* (hereinafter cited as *Walam Olum*), x.
2. Müller, *Pre-Columbian American Religions*, 162.
3. Resolution dated August 5, 1980, of the Business Committee of the Delaware Tribe of Indians meeting in Bartlesville, Oklahoma.
4. Interview with Dr. Gregory Schaaf in August 1980.
5. *Walam Olum*, 250; also see 243–268 for a description of the history of the manuscript and the original painted records.
6. Gillespie, *Dictionary of Scientific Biography*, XI, 262.
7. Malone, *Dictionary of American Biography*, XV, 323.
8. Rafinesque, *The American Nations*, 151; cf. Walam Olum, 248.
9. Rafinesque, *The American Nations*, 122–24, as reproduced in Brasseur de Bourbourg, *Quatre Lettres*, 435–437.
10. *Walam Olum*, 254–55, discusses theories about Dr. Ward's identity.
11. Squier, *Mythological Traditions*, 275, said that it had come from "the hands of the executors of the lamented Nicollet."
12. *Walam Olum*, 245–47.
13. *Walam Olum*, 246.

14. Squier, *Mythological Traditions*, 227.
15. Begley, "The First Americans," 14-20.
16. Stuart, *The Mysterious Maya*, 26.
17. Newcomb, "The Walam Olum of the Delaware Indians in Perspective," 29-32.

Chapter Two

1. Brinton, *Lenâpé and Their Legends*, 88; one of Brinton's informants recognized the language as Unalachtigo, the extinct downstream dialect of the Delaware language.
2. Penn, *Account of the Lenni Lenape*, 22.
3. Rafinesque, *The American Nations*, 124.
4. Lilly, "Pictograph Concordance with Bibliography." *Walam Olum*, 226-39; also Schaaf, "Inquiry into Parallels," 7-9.
5. *Walam Olum*, 275-77.
6. Beatty, *Journal*, 27.

Chapter Three

1. Müller, *Pre-Columbian American Religions*, 162; also Hodge, *Handbook of American Indians*, I, 385.
2. Penn, *Account of the Lenni Lenape*, 36.
3. Ibid., 30.
4. Speck, *A Study of the Delaware Big House Ceremony*, 78.
5. Müller, *Pre-Columbian American Religions*, 177; also Speck, *A Study of the Delaware Big House Ceremony*, 21, discusses the origin of the Big House.
6. Loskiel, *History of the United Brethen*, 25; cf. Squier, *Mythological Traditions*, 276.
7. Copway, *Traditional History of the Ojibway Nation*, 128, 131-32.
8. Harrington, *Dickon Among the Lenape*, 206-210.
9. Erdoes and Ortiz, 12. Retold from three 19th-century sources, including Joseph Nicolar.
10. Emerson, *Indian Myths*, 352.
11. Heckewelder, *History, Manners, and Customs*, 76.
12. Brinton, *Lenâpé and Their Legends*, 132-33.
13. Heckewelder, *History, Manners, and Customs*, 253.
14. Narrated by Kahgegahkowh (George Copway), quoted by Brinton, *American Hero-Myths*, 227-31.
15. Brinton, *Lenâpé and Their Legends*, 39-41.
16. Brennan, *American Dawn*, 180.
17. Lilly, "Pictograph Concordance with Bibliography." *Walam Olum*, 226-39; also Schaaf, "Inquiry into Parallels," 7-9.
18. Interview with Gregory Schaaf, April 11, 1979.
19. Jones, *Traditions*, Vol. I, 47-60. This legend was received by Jones himself from an aged Shawnee at Piqua in Ohio in 1823, and is also mentioned by the local Indian agent John Johnston.
20. Heckewelder, *History, Manners, and Customs*, 74.
21. Beatty, *Journal*, 91. The Moravian missionary Loskiel adds the detail that

the number of people who were left on the American shore was seven. Loskiel, *History of the United Brethen*, 24.

22. Brinton, *Lenâpé and Their Legends*, 145. Cited from Schoolcraft in *Indian Tribes*, IV: 255 (from the Shawnee in Missouri ca. 1812) and from John Johnston, Indian agent for the Shawnees, reported in *Trans. of the American Society of Antiquarians I*: 273 (from the Shawnee in Ohio ca. 1819).

23. Brinton, *Lenâpé and Their Legends*, 136–37.

24. Dusenberry, "Horn In The Ice," 12. Recorded in a personal interview with Rufus Wallowing, Lame Deer, Montana, 1955, who had heard it in 1951 from Frank Old Bird, age 80, of the Southern Cheyenne.

25. Spencer, *Indian Captivity*, 103, 128.

26. Harrington, *Religion and Ceremonies of the Lenape*, 147–51.

27. Heckewelder, "Expedition of the Lenni Lenapes." In Jones, *Traditions*, II, 156–60.

28. Heckewelder, *History, Manners, and Customs*, 47–55, as paraphrased in Squier, *Mythological Traditions*, 291–92.

Many scholars believe many aspects of Middle Mississippian Temple Mound culture show signs of influence from Mexican or Mesoamerican sources. Although the Talegas were actually a Native American culture, some authors have speculated that the Moundbuilders were wandering Celts, or Phoenician explorers, or a colony of Romans. The Book of Morman is supposed to have been a repository of ancient wisdom left by one of the last of the Moundbuilders, the descendants of the Lost Tribes of Israel, before they were wiped out by hordes of barbarian invaders, like the fall of Rome at the beginning of the Dark Ages. But as the archeologist Brian Fagan says:

> whatever one's views on the theological controversies around the Book of Mormon, the existence of the victims of these great wars, frequently amounting to tens of thousands, was verified by the hundreds of recorded instances of skeletons coming to light as mounds were excavated by treasure hunters or razed by the plow. (Fagan, *Elusive Treasure*, 118.)

29. See note 28.

30. Adams, *Legends of the Delaware Indians and Picture Writing*, 39–44, 34, 70–71.

31. Heckewelder, *History, Manners, and Customs*, 49–53, as paraphrased in Squier, *Mythological Traditions*, 291–92.

32. Weslager, *The Delaware Indians: A History*, 43–47.

33. Brinton, *Lenape and Their Legends*, 36.

34. Heckewelder, *History, Manners, and Customs*, 55, as paraphrased in Squier, *Mythological Traditions*, 292.

Chapter Four

1. Erdoes and Ortiz, *American Indian Myths and Legends*, 76.

2. Brinton, *Lenâpé and Their Legends*, 100, 126.

3. Copway, *Traditional History of the Ojibway Nation*, 132; also in Müller, *Pre-Columbian American Religions*, 175.

4. Brinton and Anthony, A *Lenape-English Dictionary*, 73. Anthony notes that it connotes more of a spirit than a creator.

5. Harrington, "Vestiges of Material Culture," 415.

6. Müller, *Pre-Columbian American Religions*, 170.

7. Brinton, *Lenâpé and Their Legends*, 135-36.

8. Heckewelder, *History, Manners and Customs*, 76.

9. Brinton, *Lenâpé and Their Legends*, 39-41.

10. Narrated by Kahgegahkowh (George Copway), quoted by Brinton, *American Hero-Myths*, 227-31.

11. Treistman, *Prehistory of China*, 8-9.

12. Genet, *Ancient China*, 30, 38.

13. Treistman, *Prehistory of China*, 18-19, fn.1

14. Ibid., 26-30.

15. Ibid., 31-32.

16. Hirth, *Ancient History of China*, 13, 66.

17. Giddings, *Ancient Men of the Arctic*, 44, 149, 212.

18. Kopper, *Smithsonian Book of North American Indians*, 99-105. Also Giddings, *Ancient Men of the Arctic*, 242.

19. Loskiel, *History of the United Brethen*, 29, describes how the Delawares counted using a decimal system.

20. See Penn, *Account of the Lenni Lenape*, 35-39, for an excellent description of their leaders in council.

21. Waldman, *Atlas of the North American Indian*, 64.

22. Goodman, *American Genesis*, 51.

23. "Pomatare, the Flying Beaver" in Jones, *Traditions*, I, 57. Jones himself received this story from an aged Shawnee near Piqua, Ohio, in 1823.

24. Burland, *Mythology of the Americas*, 26.

25. Harrington, *Religion and Ceremonies of the Lenape*, 147-51.

26. Cheng-Mei Chang, "Chinese Writing - A System of Characters Rich in Cultural Diversity," 45.

27. Pilling, "Yurok," 137; also Sapir, "Wiyot and Yurok, Algonquin Languages of California," 617-46.

28. Heckewelder, *History, Manners, and Customs*, 30.

29. See Grinnell, *Blackfoot Lodge Tales*; Ahenakew, *Voices of the Plains Cree*; and Seger, *Early Days Among the Cheyenne and Arapahoe Indians*.

30. Wedel, *Prehistoric Man on the Great Plains*, 255-7.

31. Grinnell, *Blackfoot Lodge Tales*, 230, gives a description of an ancient buffalo drive.

32. Collier, *Indians of the Americans*, 94, lists the ingenious variety of uses for the parts of a buffalo.

33. *Walam Olum*, 279.

34. Heckewelder, "The Expedition of the Lenni Lenape." In Jones, *Traditions*, II, 156-160.

35. Wedel, *Prehistoric Man on the Great Plains*, 35.

36. Weslager, *The Delaware Indians: A History*, 88. A picture of Cahokia in its prime is in Maxwell, ed., *America's Fascinating Indian Heritage*, 100.

37. Cahokia staff archeologist Bill Iseminger in *Los Angeles Times*, April 4, 1991, A5.

38. Jones, *Traditions*, II, 163, and separately in Heckewelder, *History, Manners, and Customs*, 28.

39. Josephy, ed., *American Heritage Book of Indians*, 147-52; contains a full description of the Natchez.
40. Morgan, *Fort Ancient*, 26. The estimated date of this fortress is 1000 A. D.
41. Heckewelder, *History, Manners, and Customs*, 220.
42. Heckewelder, "The Fall of the Lenape." Jones, *Traditions*, I, 87.
43. Josephy, ed. *American Heritage Book of Indians*, 161.
44. Beatty, *Journal*, 27.
45. Ibid.
46. Brinton, *Lenâpé and Their Legends*, 145.
47. Ibid., 137.
48. Tooker, "The League of the Iroquois: Its History, Politics and Ritual," *Handbook of North American Indians*, Vol. 15: *Northeast*, 427.
49. Brinton, *Lenâpé and Their Legends*, 132.
50. Brasser, "Early Indian-American Contacts," 78-88.
51. Weslager, *The Delaware Indians, A History*, 43-47; Brinton, *Lenape and Their Legends*, 36.
52. Barbour, *Pocahontas*, 12-20, 50.
53. Heckewelder, *History, Manners, and Customs*, xli; cf. Weslager, *The Delaware Indians, A History*, 47, n. 1.
54. Jones, *Traditions*, II, 158.
55. Lipinsky, *Giovanni da Verrazzano*, 12-13.
56. Also see Heckewelder, "Indian Tradition of the First Arrival of the Dutch at Manhattan Island, Now New-York," 70-73, a less polished version of this story that is based on the notes Heckewelder took on the spot during the original recitation "by aged and respected Delawares, Monseys and Mahicanni [Mohicans]" around 1762.

Part Three: The Strangers

Chapter Five

1. Grumet, *The Lenapes*, 33-34.
2. Weslager, *The Delaware Indians, A History*, 118, 124-27.
3. Ibid., 161.
4. Heckewelder, *History, Manners, and Customs*, 34.
5. Weslager, *The Delaware Indians, A History*, 180-81.
6. Grumet, *The Lenapes*, 43.
7. Weslager, *The Delaware Indians, A History*, 187-90.
8. Ibid., 168-169, 175.
9. Ibid., 177.
10. Ibid., 178, 193, 234-39.
11. Ibid., 245.
12. de Schweinitz, *Life and Times of David Zeisberger*, 444; cf. Brinton, *Lenâpé and Their Legends*, 113.
13. See Schaaf's *Wampum Belts and Peace Trees*, which is based on a previously unknown cache of documents by the American Indian agent George Morgan.
14. Weslager, *The Delaware Indians: A History*, 305.
15. Ibid., 298-99.
16. Ibid., 298-99.

17. Ibid., 315–17.
18. Ibid., 322.
19. Ibid., 335.
20. Ibid., 329.
21. Ibid., 352.

Chapter Six

1. Irving, *Western Journals of Washington Irving*, 164.
2. Irving, *Indian Sketches*, 242.
3. Adams, *A Brief History*, 34; cf. Weslager, *The Delaware Indians, A History*, 380.
4. Dodge, *Our Wild Indians*, 554.
5. Grumet, *The Lenapes*, 100.

Chapter Seven

1. "Ubar, Fabled Lost City, Found by L.A. Team." *Los Angeles Times*, Feb. 5, 1992, A1.
2. Osborne, *Mythology of the Americans*, 289.
3. Stuart, *The Mysterious Maya*, 95.
4. Gasselin, *Les Sauvages du Mississippi*, I, 31–51.
5. Copway, *Traditional History*, 129.
6. Penn, *Account of the Lenni Lenape*, 55–56.
7. Brinton, *Lenâpé and Their Legends*, 145, n. 2.
8. de Acosta, *Natural and Moral History of the Indies*, I, 25.
9. Osborne, *Mythology of the Americas*, 317.
10. Collier, *Indians of the Americas* 101.

Bibliography

(* indicates works of special value relating to the Lenni Lenape or Delawares)

General Native American History and Prehistory

Begley, Sharon. "The First Americans," *Newsweek* Special Issue (1991): 14–20.

Brennan, Louis A. *American Dawn: A New Model of American Prehistory.* London: Collier-Macmillan, Ltd., 1970

Burland, Cottie, Irene Nicholson, and Harold Osborne. *Mythology of the Americas.* London: Hambyn Publishing Group, 1970.

Cienza de León, Pedro de. *The Travels of Pedro de Cienza de León, Contained in the First Part of His Chronicle of Peru, AD 1532–1550.* London: Hukluyt Society. No. 33. London, 1864.

Claiborne, Robert. *The First Americans.* New York: Time-Life Books, 1973.

Collier, John. *Indians of the Americas: The Long Hope.* New York: Norton, 1947.

Fagan, Brian. *Elusive Treasure: The Story of Early Archeologists in the Americas.* New York: Charles Scribner's Sons, 1977.

——. "Who Were The Mound Builders?" In *Mysteries of the Past,* edited by Joseph J. Thorndike, Jr. New York: American Heritage Publishing Co., Inc., 1977.

Franglin, Paula Angle. *Indians of North America: The Eight Culture Areas and How Their Inhabitants Lived Before the Coming of the Whites.* New York: McKay, 1979.

Gallatin, Albert. *A Synopsis of the Indian Tribes Within the United States East of the Rocky Mountains, and in the British and Russian Possessions in North America.* Transactions and Collections of the American Antiquarian Society 2 (1836). Reprint. New York: AMS Press, 1973.

Gasselin, M. L'Abbe Amédée, *Les Sauvages du Mississippi (1698–1708).* 2 vols. Quebec: 15th International Congress of Americanists, 1906.

Goodman, Jeffrey. *American Genesis: The American Indian and the Origins of Modern Man.* New York: Summit Books, 1981.

Grant, Bruce. *The American Indian, Yesterday and Today: A Profusely Illustrated Encyclopedia of the American Indian.* New York: Dutton, 1955.

Hodge, Frederick Webb. *Handbook of American Indians North of Mexico.* Washington, D.C.: Government Printing Office, 1910.

Huntington, Ellsworth. *Red Man's Continent: A Chronicle of Aboriginal America.* New Haven: Yale University Press, 1920.

Jennings, Francis. *The Invasion of America: Indians, Colonialism and the Cant of Conquest.* Chapel Hill: University of North Carolina Press, 1975.

Jennings, Jesse D. *The Prehistory of North America.* New York: McGraw-Hill, 1968.

Josephy, Alvin M., ed. *The American Heritage Book of Indians.* New York: American Heritage Publishing Co., 1961.

Kopper, Philip. *The Smithsonian Book of North American Indians.* Washington, D.C.: Smithsonian Books, 1986.

La Farge, Oliver. *A Pictorial History of the American Indian.* New York: Crown Publishers, 1956.

Leonard, Jonathan N. *Ancient America.* New York: Time-Life Books, 1973.

LePoer, Barbara A. *Chronology of the American Indian.* St. Clair Shores, MI: Scholarly Press, 1975.

———. *A Concise Dictionary of Indian Tribes of North America.* Edited by Kendall T. LePoer. Algonac, MI: Reference Publications Inc., 1979.

Macneish, Richard S., comp. *Early Man in America: Readings From "Scientific American."* San Francisco: W.H. Freeman, 1973.

Mallery, Garrick. *Picture-Writing of the American Indians.* Vol. 1. Washington, D.C., 1988. Reprint. New York: Dover Publications, 1972.

Martin, Paul Sidney. *Indians Before Columbus: Twenty Thousand Years of North American History Revealed by Archeology.* Chicago: University of Chicago Press, 1947.

Maxwell, James A., ed. *America's Fascinating Indian Heritage.* Pleasantville, NY: Reader's Digest Association, 1978.

McKusick, Marshall. *Men of Ancient Iowa, as Revealed by Archeological Discoveries.* Ames, IA: Iowa State University Press, 1964.

McNickle, D'Arcy. *They Came Here First: The Epic of the American Indian.* Philadelphia: J.B. Lippencott, 1949.

Morgan, Richard G. *Fort Ancient.* Columbus: Ohio Historical Society, 1965.

Nichols, Frances S. [Gaither], comp. *Index to Schoolcraft's "Indian Tribes of the United States."* Washington, D.C.: U.S. Government Printing Office, 1954.

Page, Evelyn. *American Genesis: Pre-colonial Writing in the North.* Boston: Gambit, 1973.

Palmer, Rose Amelia. *The North American Indians: An Account of the American Indians North of Mexico, Compiled From the Original Sources.* Washington, D.C.: Smithsonian Institution, 1934.

Porter, C. Fayne. *Our Indian Heritage: Profiles of 12 Great Leaders.* Philadelphia: Chilton Book Company, 1964.

Reed, Nelson, John W. Bennett, and James W. Porter. "Solid Core Drilling of Monk's Mound; Technique and Findings." *American Antiquities* 33, no. 2 (1968): 137–148.

Sale, Kirkpatrick. *The Conquest of Paradise: Christopher Columbus and the Columbian Legacy.* New York: Alfred A. Knopf, 1990.

Schoolcraft, Henry Rowe. *History of the Indian Tribes of the United States: Their Present Condition and Prospects, and a Sketch of Their Ancient Status.* Washington, D.C.: Lippencott & Co., 1857.

Schwartz, Douglas W. *Conceptions of Kentucky Prehistory.* Lexington, KY: University of Kentucky Press, 1967,

Silverberg, Robert. *Home of the Red Man: Indian North America Before Columbus*. New York: New York Graphic Society, 1963.

Spencer, Robert F., and Jesse D. Jennings. *Native Americans: Prehistory and Ethnology of the North American Indians*. New York: Harper & Row, 1977.

Stuart, George E., and Gene S. Stuart. *The Mysterious Maya*. Washington, D.C.: National Geographic Society, 1977.

Tocqueville, Alexis de. *Democracy in America*. Translated by Henry Reeve. New York, 1840. Reprint, edited by Phillips Bradley. New York: Alfred A. Knopf, 1985.

Waldman, Carl. *Atlas of the North American Indian*. Illustrated by Molly Braun. New York: Facts on File Publications, 1985.

Walking Turtle, Eagle. *Indian America: A Traveler's Companion*. Santa Fe, NM: John Muir Publications, 1991.

Washburn, Wilcomb E. *The Indian of America*. New York: Harper & Row, 1975.

Wedel, Waldo R. *Prehistoric Man on the Great Plains*. Norman, OK: University of Oklahoma Press, 1961.

Werner, M.R. *Tammany Hall*. Garden City, NY: Doubleday, Doran & Company, Inc., 1928.

Lenape (Algonquian-Speaking) Tribes Related to the Lenni Lenape or Delawares

Ahenakew, Edward. *Voices of the Plains Cree*. Toronto: McClelland & Stewart, 1973.

Catlin, George. *Letters and Notes on the Manners, Customs and Condition of the North American Indians, Written During Eight Years' Travel Among the Wildest Tribes of Indians in North America in 1832, 33, 34, 35, 36, 37, 38, and 39*. London, 1841. Reprint. Minneapolis: Ross & Haines, 1965.

Cook, Sherburne. *The Indian Population of New England in the Seventeenth Century*. Berkeley: University of California Press, 1976.

Copway, George [Kahgegahkowh]. *The Life History and Travels of Kah-ge-gah-kowh (George Copway), a Young Indian Chief of the Ojibwa Nation, a Convert to the Christian Faith, and a Missionary to His People for Twelve Years*. Philadelphia: James Harmstead: 1847.

———. *The Traditional History and Characteristic Sketches of the Ojibway*

Nation. London: Charles Gilpin, 1850.

Flannery, Regina. *An Analysis of Coastal Algonquin Culture.* Washington, D.C.: Catholic University of America Press, 1939.

Goddard, Ives. "Central Algonquian Languages," In *Handbook of North American Indians.* Vol. 15, *Northeast.* Edited by Bruce G. Trigger, 583–587. Washington, D.C.: Smithsonian Institution, 1978.

Hyde, George E. *Indians of the Woodlands: From Prehistoric Times to 1725.* Norman: University of Oklahoma Press, 1962.

Kinietz, Vernon. *The Indians of the Western Great Lakes.* Ann Arbor, MI: University of Michigan Press, 1940.

Mowat, Farley. *People of the Deer.* Boston: Little, Brown & Co., 1952.

Pilling, Arnold R. Yurok." In *Handbook of North American Indians.* Vol. 8, *California.* Edited by William C. Sturtevant. Washington, D.C.: Smithsonian Institution, 1978.

Salomon, Julian Harris. *Indians of the Lower Hudson Region: The Munsee.* New City, NY: Historical Society of Rockland County, 1982.

Sapir, Edward. "Wiyot and Yurok, Algonkin Languages of California." *American Anthropologist* 15, no. 4 (1975): 617–46.

Schaffer, Claude E. *Blackfoot Shaking Tent.* Calgary: Glenbow-Alberta Institute, 1969.

Seger, John H. *Early Days Among the Cheyenne and Arapahoe Indians.* Norman, OK: University of Oklahoma Press, 1934.

Siegel, Beatrice. *Indians of the Woodland, Before and After the Pilgrims.* Boston: Walker, 1972.

Speck, Frank G. *Naskapi: The Savage Hunters of the Labrador Peninsula.* Norman, Oklahoma: University of Oklahoma Press, 1935.

Spencer, Joab [Reverend Charles Bluejacket]. "The Shawnee Indians." *Transactions of the Kansas State Historical Society* 10 (1908): 382–402.

Tanner, John. *A Narrative of the Captivity and Adventures of John Tanner (U.S. Interpreter at the Saut de Ste. Marie) During Thirty Years' Residence Among the Indians.* Philadelphia, 1830. Reprint, edited by Edwin James. Minneapolis: Ross & Haines, 1956.

Trigger, Bruce G. "Cultural Unity and Diversity." In *Handbook of North American Indians.* Vol. 15, *Northeast.* Edited by Bruce G. Trigger, 798–804. Washington, D.C.: Smithsonian Institution, 1978.

Weslager, C.A. *Delaware's Forgotten Folk: The Story of the Moors and Nanticokes.* Philadelphia: University of Pennsylvania Press, 1943.

General Lenape Family (Algonquian) Mythology and Legends

Alexander, Hartley Burr. *Mythology of All Races.* Vol. 10. Boston: Archeological Institute of America, 1965.

——. *The World's Rim: Great Mysteries of the North American Indians.* Lincoln, NE: University of Nebraska Press, 1967.

Bloomfield, Leonard. *Sacred Stories of the Sweet Grass Cree.* Ottawa: F.A. Acland, 1930.

Brandon, William. *The Magic World: American Indian Songs and Poems.* New York: Morrow & Co., 1971.

Brinton, Daniel G. *The Myths of the New World: A Treatise on the Symbolism and Mythology of the Red Race of America.* New York: Henry Holt & Co., 1876.

——. *American Hero-myths.* Philadelphia: H.C. Watts & Co., 1882.

——. *Aboriginal American Authors and Their Productions, Especially Those in the Native Languages: A Chapter in the History of Literature.* Philadelphia, 1883. Reprint. Chicago: Checagou Reprints, 1970.

Clark, Ella Elizabeth. *Indian Legends from the Northern Rockies.* Norman, OK: University of Oklahoma Press, 1966.

Curtin, Jeremiah. *Creation Myths of Primitive America.* Boston: Little, Brown & Co., 1903.

Dusenberry, Verne. "Horn in the Ice: An Introduction to the Earliest Cheyennes." In *Red Man's West: True Stories of the Frontier Indians from MONTANA, the Magazine of Western History.* Edited by Michael S. Kennedy, 11–20. New York: Hastings House, 1965.

Erdoes, Richard, and Alfonso Ortiz, eds. *American Indian Myths and Legends.* New York: Pantheon Books, 1984.

Grinell, George Bird. *Blackfoot Lodge Tales: The Story of a Prairie People.* Corner House Publishers, 1892. Reprint. Lincoln, NE: University of Nebraska Press, 1962.

Howard, James H. *Shawnee! The Ceremonialism of a Native American Tribe and Its Cultural Background.* Athens, OH: Ohio University Press, 1981.

Kinietz, Vernon, and Erminie W. Voegelin, eds. *Shawnee Traditions: C.C. Trowbridge's Account.* Ann Arbor: University of Michigan Museum of Anthropology, Occasional Contributions 9, 1939.

*Leland, Charles G. *The Algonquin Legends of New England*. Boston: Houghton, Mifflin, 1884.

Marriott, Alice, and Carol K. Rachlin. *American Indian Mythology*. New York: Thomas Y. Crowell Co., 1968.

*Müller, Werner. "Supreme Being and Big House: The Delaware and Algonquian of the Atlantic Seaboard." In *Pre-Columbian American Religions*. Translated by Stanley Davis. New York: Holt Rinehart and Winston, 1968.

Sanders, Thomas Edward, and Walter W. Peek. *Literature of the American Indian*. Beverly Hills: Glencoe, 1973.

Schultz, James Willard. *Blackfeet Tales of Glacier National Park*. Boston and New York: Houghton Mifflin Company, 1916.

Spencer, Joab [Reverend Charles Bluejacket]. "Shawnee Folklore." *Journal of American Folklore* 22 (1909): 319–29.

Squier, Ephraim George. *The Serpent Symbol and the Worship of the Reciprocal Principles in Nature in America*. New York: G.P. Putnam, 1851.

Lenni Lenape (Delaware) Traditions, Legends and Language

*Adams, Richard C. *The Ancient Religion of the Delaware Indians and Observations and Reflections*. Washington, D.C.: Law Reporter Printing Co., 1904.

*——. *Legends of the Delaware Indians and Picture Writing*. Washington, D.C.: 1905.

——. *The Adoption of Mew-seu-qua, Tecumseh's Father, and the Philosophy of the Delaware Indians, with Unpolished Gems*. Washington, D.C.: Crane Printing Co., 1917.

Brinton, Daniel G. "Lenape Conversations." *Journal of American Folklore* 1 (1888): 38–39.

*Brinton, Daniel G., and Reverend A.S. Anthony. *A Lenâpé-English Dictionary*. The Pennsylvania Students' Series, vol. I. Philadelphia: The Historical Society of Pennsylvania, 1888.

Dean, Nora Thompson, and Jay Miller. "A Personal Account of the Unami Delaware Big House Rite." *Pennsylvania Archeologist* (1977): 39–43.

*Emerson, Ellen Russell. *Indian Myths*. Minneapolis: Ross & Haines, 1925.

Goddard, Ives. "Delaware." In *Handbook of North American Indians*.

Vol. 15, *Northeast*. Edited by Bruce G. Trigger, 213–239. Washington, D.C.: Smithsonian Institution, 1978.

——. "Eastern Algonquian Languages." In *Handbook of North American Indians*. Vol. 15, *Northeast*. Edited by Bruce G. Trigger, 70–77. Washington, D.C.: Smithsonian Institution.

Harrington, Mark R. "Vestiges of Material Culture Among the Canadian Delawares." *American Anthropologist* 10 (1908): 415.

——. "A Preliminary Sketch of Lenape Culture." *American Anthropologist* 15, no. 5, (1913): 234.

*——. *Religion and Ceremonies of the Lenape*. New York: Museum of the American Indian, Heye Foundation, 1921.

——. *Dickon Among the Lenape Indians*. Philadelphia & Chicago: The John C. Winston Company, 1938. (Reprinted as *The Indians of New Jersey, Dickon Among the Lenapes*. New Brunswick, NJ: Rutgers University Press, 1963.)

Heckewelder, Reverend John. "The Expedition of the Lenni Lenape." *Transactions of the American Philosophical Society* 1 (1799): 54–74.

*——. *An Account of the History, Manners and Customs of the Indian Nations Who Once Inhabited Pennsylvania and the Neighboring States*. Philadelphia, 1818. Reprint. Philadelphia: Memoirs of the Historical Society of Pennsylvania, no. 12, 1876.

——. "Indian Tradition of the First Arrival of the Dutch at Manhattan Island, Now New-York." *Collections of the New York Historical Society*, series 2, vol. 1 (1841): 70–73.

*Jones, James Athearn. *Traditions of the North American Indians*. Vols. I–III. London, 1829. Reprint. Upper Saddle River, NJ: Literature House/Gregg Press, 1970.

Kinietz, Vernon. *Delaware Culture Chronology*. Indianapolis: Indiana Historical Society, 1946.

Miller, Jay. "Delaware Language and Culture." In *Papers of the 1978 Mid-America Linguistics Conference at Oklahoma*, eds. Ralph E. Cooley, Mervin R. Barnes, and John A. Dunn. 32–31.

Penn, William. *William Penn's Own Account of the Lenni Lenape or Delaware Indians*. Revised and edited by Albert Cook Myers. Somerset, NJ: Middle Atlantic Press, 1970.

*Speck, Frank G. *A Study of the Delaware Big House Ceremony*. Harrisburg, PA: Publications of the Pennsylvania Historical Commission 2, 1931.

*——. "Oklahoma Delaware Ceremonial Feasts and Dances." *Memoirs of the American Philosophical Society*, no. 7, 1937.

—— with Jesse Moses. *The Celestial Bear Comes Down To Earth.* Reading, PA: Scientific Publications 7, Reading Public Museum and Art Gallery, 1945.

Trowbridge, Charles C. "Tradition of the Lenape Lenaupee or Delawares" and (c. 1824) "Delaware Grammar." C.C. Trowbridge Papers. Michigan Historical Collections, University of Michigan, Ann Arbor.

Weslager, C.A. "A New Look at Brinton's Lenape-English Dictionary." *Pennsylvania Archeologist* 42, no. 4 (1972).

Wilcox, Frank Nelson. *Ohio Indian Trails: A Pictorial Survey of the Indian Trails of Ohio.* Edited by William A. McGill. Kent, OH: Kent State University Press, 1970.

Zeisberger, David. *Zeisberger's Indian Dictionary, English, German, Iroquois–the Onondaga and Algonquin–the Delaware: Printed From the Original Manuscript in Harvard College Library.* Cambridge, MA: J. Wilson & Son, 1887.

Delaware Indian History (1492–Present)

*Adams, Richard C. "A Brief History of the Delaware Indians." *Congressional Record.* 59th Cong., 1st sess., 1906.

Barbour, Philip L. *Pocahontas and Her World: A Chronicle of America's First Settlement in Which is Related the Story of the Indians and the Englishmen, Particularly Captain John Smith, Captain Samuel Argall, and Master John Rolfe.* Boston: Houghton Mifflin, 1970.

Beatty, Charles. *Journals of Charles Beatty 1762–1769.* London, 1768. Reprint. University Park: Pennsylvania State University Press, 1962.

——. *The Journal of a Two Month's Tour With a View of Promoting Religion Among the Frontier Inhabitants of Pennsylvania and of Introducing Christianity Among the Indians to the Westward of the Alegh-geny Mountains.* London: W. Davenhill and G. Pearch, 1768.

Brasser, T.J. "Early Indian-American Contacts." In *Handbook of North American Indians.* Vol. 15, *Northeast.* Edited by Bruce G. Trigger, 78–88. Washington, D.C.: Smithsonian Institution, 1978.

Dodge, Richard Irving. *Our Wild Indians: Thirty-three Years' Personal Experience Among the Red Men of the Great West.* Hartford, CT: A.D. Worthington and Co., 1882.

Fliegel, Reverend Carl John, ed. *Index to the Records of the Moravian Mission Among the Indians of North America.* New Haven, CT: Research Publications, 1970.

Grumet, Robert S. *The Lenapes.* Edited by Frank W. Porter III. New York: Chelsea House Publishers, 1989.

Heckewelder, Reverend John. *Narrative of the Mission of the United Brethren Among the Delaware and Mohegan Indians, From its Commencement in the Year 1740 to the Close in the Year 1808.* Philadelphia: 1820. Reprint. New York: Arno Press and the New York Times, 1971.

Huebner, Francis C. *Charles Killbuck, An Indian's Story of the Border Wars of the American Revolution.* Washington, D.C.: Herbert Publishing Co., 1902.

Irving, John Treat, Jr. *Indian Sketches, Taken During an Expedition to the Pawnee Tribes.* Philadelphia: Carey, Lea and Blanchard, 1835. Reprint, edited by John Francis McDermott. Norman, OK: University of Oklahoma Press, 1955.

Irving, Washington. *Western Journals of Washington Irving.* New York, 1834. Reprint, edited by John Francis McDermott. Norman: University of Oklahoma Press, 1944.

Lipinsky, Lino S. *Giovanni da Verrazzano, the Discoverer of New York Bay, 1524: A Graphic Documentation of the Discoveries by the Great Florentine Explorer and Humanist of the Renaissance.* New York: Museum of the City of New York and the Instuto Italiano di Cultura in New York City, 1958.

Long, John. *Voyages and Travels of an Indian Interpreter and Trader, Describing the Manners and Customs of the North American Indians.* London, 1791. Reprint. New York: Johnson Reprint Co., 1968.

Loskiel, George Henry. *History of the Mission of the United Brethren Among the Indians of North America.* Translated by Christian Ignatius La Trobe. London: Brethren's Society for the Furtherance of the Gospel, 1794.

Martin, Calvin. *Keepers of the Game: Indian-animal Relationships and the Fur Trade.* Berkeley: University of California Press, 1978.

Morgan, Lewis Henry. *League of the Ho-de'-no-sau-nee or Iroquois.* New York: Dodd, Mead and Company, 1901.

Powers, Mabel [Yehsonnohwehs]. *The Indian as Peacemaker.* New York: Fleming H. Revell Company, 1932.

Schaaf, Gregory. *Wampum Belts and Peace Trees: George Morgan, Native Americans and Revolutionary Diplomacy.* Golden, CO: Fulcrum Publishing, 1990.

Schweinitz, Edmund Alexander de. *The Life and Times of David Zeisberger, the Western Pioneer and Apostle to the Indians.* Philadelphia: J.B. Lippencott, 1870. Reprint. New York: Arno Press and The New York Times, 1971.

Shaw, Charles. *Indian Life in Texas.* Austin: State House Press, 1987.

Smith, Samuel. *The Colonial History of New Jersey.* Burlington, NJ: 1765. Reprint. Trenton, NJ: W.S. Sharp, 1890.

Spencer, Oliver M. *The Indian Captivity of O.M. Spencer.* Philadelphia, 1834. Reprint, edited by Milo M. Quaife. Chicago: R.R. Donnelley, 1917.

Tooker, Elisabeth. "The League of the Iroquois: Its History, Politics and Ritual." In *Handbook of North American Indians.* Vol. 15, *Northeast.* Edited by Bruce G. Trigger, 418–441. Washington, D.C.: Smithsonian Institution, 1978.

Wallace, Anthony F.C. *King of the Delawares: Teedyuscung.* Philadelphia: University of Pennsylvania Press, 1949.

Weslager, C.A. *The Delaware Indians: A History.* New Brunswick, NJ: Rutgers University Press, 1972.

———. *The Delaware Westward Migration, With Texts of Two Manuscripts, 1821–22, Responding to General Lewis Cass' Inquiries About Lenape Culture and Language.* Wallingford, PA: Middle Atlantic Press, 1978.

———. *The Delawares, A Critical Bibliography.* Bloomington, IN: Indiana University Press, 1978.

Studies or Publications of the Wallam Olum or Red Record

Barlow, William, and David O. Powell. "'The Late Dr. Ward of Indiana': Rafinesque's Source of the Walam Olum." *Indiana Magazine of History* 82, no. 2 (1986): 185–193.

Boewe, Charles. "A Note on Rafinesque, the Walam Olum, the Book of Mormon, and the Mayan Glyphs." *Numen* 32, no. 1 (1985): 101–113.

———. "The Walam Olum and Dr. Ward, Again." *Indiana Magazine of History* 83, no. 4 (1987): 344–359.

Brasseur de Bourbourg, Charles Etienne, *Quatre Lettres sur le Mexique, exposition absolue du Systeme Hieroglyphique Mexicain . . .* Paris: Auguste

Durand et Pedone, 1868. (Rafinesque's first publication of the Wallam Olum is reproduced on 435–448.)

*Brinton, Daniel G. *The Lenâpé and Their Legends, With the Complete Text and Symbols of the Walam Olum, a New Translation, and an Inquiry Into Its Authenticity*. New York: AMS Press, 1884.

Hoffman, Daniel. *Brotherly Love*. New York: Vintage, 1981.

*Indiana Historical Society. *Walam Olum or Red Score: The Migration Legend of the Lenni Lenape or Delaware Indians—A New Translation, Interpreted by Linguistic, Historical, Archeological, Ethnological, and Physical Anthropological Studies*. Chicago: The Lakeside Press, 1954.

Lilly, Eli. "Tentative Speculations on the Chronology of the Walam Olum and the Migration Route of the Lenape." *Proceedings of the Indiana Academy of Science* 54 (1944): 33.

Madison, James H. *Eli Lilly, A Life, 1885–1977*. Indianapolis: Indiana Historical Society, 1989.

Mahr, August C. "Walam Olum I,17: A Proof of Rafinesque's Integrity." *American Anthropologist* 59 (1957): 705–708.

Newcomb, William B. "The Walam Olum of the Delaware Indians in Perspective." *Texas Journal of Science* 7, no. 1 (1955): 57–63. Reprint. *Bulletin of the Archeological Society of New Jersey* 30 (1974): 29–32.

Norwood, Joseph White. *The Tammany Legend (Tamanend)*. Boston: Meador Publishing Co., 1938.

Rafinesque, Constantine S. *The American Nations; or, Outlines of Their General History, Ancient and Modern*. Philadelphia: C.S. Rafinesque, 1836.

Rothenburg, Jerome, and George Quasha. *America: A Prophecy*. New York: Random House, 1973.

*Squier, Ephraim George. "Historical and Mythological Traditions of the Algonquins, with a Translation of the Walam-Olum, or Bark Record of the Lenni-Lenape." *American Review* (Feb., 1849): 273–293.

Velie, Alan R., ed. *American Indian Literature: An Anthology*. Norman and London: University of Oklahoma Press, 1991.

Zolla, Elemire. *The Writer and the Shaman: A Morphology of the American Indian*. New York: Harcourt Brace, 1973.

Ancient Chinese and Arctic Region Studies

Genet, Jacques. *Ancient China From the Beginnings to the Empire.*

Translated by Raymond Rudorff. Berkeley: University of California Press, 1968.

Giddings, J. Louis. *Ancient Men of the Arctic*. New York: Alfred A. Knopf, 1967.

Hirth, Friederich. *The Ancient History of China*. New York, 1908. Reprint. New York: Books for Libraries Press, 1969.

Ho, Ping-ti. *The Cradle of the East: An Inquiry Into the Indigenous Origins of Techniques and Ideas of Neolithic and Early-historic China, 5000–1000 BC*. Hong Kong: Chinese University of Hong Kong, and Chicago: University of Chicago Press, 1975.

Hopkins, David M., ed. *The Bering Land Bridge*. Stanford: Stanford University Press, 1967.

Hunt, William R. *Arctic Passage: The Turbulent History of the Land and People of the Bering Sea 1697–1975*. New York: Scribner & Sons, 1975.

Levenson, Joseph Richmond, and Franz Scurmann. *China: An Interpretive History, From the Beginnings to the Fall of Han*. Berkeley: University of California Press, 1969.

Poncins, Gontran de. *Kabloona*. New York: Reynal & Hitchcock, 1941.

Ssu-ma, Ch'ien. *Records of the Historian: Chapters From the Shih Chi*. Translated by Burton Watson. New York: Columbia University Press, 1969.

Treistman, Judith M. *The Prehistory of China: An Archeological Exploration*. Garden City, NY: Natural History Press, 1972.

Studies on the Origins of Sacred and Historical Texts

Bloom, Harold. *The Book of J*. Translated by David Rosenberg. New York: Vintage Books, 1990.

Claiborne, Robert. *The Birth of Writing*. New York: Time-Life Books, 1974.

Farris, G.J. "Recognizing Indian Folk History as Real History: A Fort Ross Example." *American Indian Quarterly* 13 (1989): 471–80.

Ferro, Marc. *The Use and Abuse of History, or, How the Past Is Taught*. Paris: Payot, 1981. Reprint and Translation. London: Routledge & Kegan Paul, 1984.

Jones, Gwyn. *The Norse Atlantic Saga, Being the Norse Voyages of Discovery and Settlement to Iceland, Greenland, and America*. London &

New York: Oxford University Press, 1964.

Krupat, Arnold. *For Those Who Come After: A Study of Native American Autobiography.* Berkeley: University of California Press, 1985.

Mutwa, Vasamazulu Credo. *Indaba, My Children.* London: Kahn & Averill, 1966.

Index